Studies in Early Medicine 1

Series Editors: Sally Crawford and Christina Lee

Bodies of Knowledge: Cultural Interpretations of Illness and Medicine in Medieval Europe

Edited by

Sally Crawford
Christina Lee

BAR International Series 2170
2010

Published in 2016 by
BAR Publishing, Oxford

BAR International Series 2170

Studies in Early Medicine 1
Bodies of Knowledge: Cultural Interpretations of Illness and Medicine in Medieval Europe

ISBN 978 1 4073 0714 5

BAR Publishing is the trading name of British Archaeological Reports (Oxford) Ltd. British Archaeological Reports was first incorporated in 1974 to publish the BAR Series, International and British. In 1992 Hadrian Books Ltd became part of the BAR group. This volume was originally published by Archaeopress in conjunction with British Archaeological Reports (Oxford) Ltd / Hadrian Books Ltd, the Series principal publisher, in 2010. This present volume is published by BAR Publishing, 2016.

Printed in England

BAR
PUBLISHING

BAR titles are available from:

BAR Publishing
122 Banbury Rd, Oxford, OX2 7BP, UK
EMAIL info@barpublishing.com
PHONE +44 (0)1865 310431
FAX +44 (0)1865 316916
www.barpublishing.com

Foreword

Studies in Early Medicine originated in a series of workshops on 'Disease and Disability in Early Medieval Europe' organised jointly by Sally Crawford and Christina Lee, with support from Robert Arnott, and held at the Universities of Birmingham, Nottingham and Oxford from 2005-2009. The *Disease and Disability* workshops were intended as an interdisciplinary forum for those working in the field of early medieval attitudes to disease, health and medicine. Those who attended included archaeologists, historians, literary scholars and medical professionals, some of whom were medical specialists, and some who were researchers whose more usual range of interests had intersected with the topic of early medieval disease and disability. It quickly became apparent that there was a wider range of interest, beyond the boundaries of the medieval world, in perceptions of health and disease in the past. Discussions at the last *Disease and Disability* workshop focussed on the need for a publication which would allow research in different disciplines – archaeology, medicine, philosophy, linguistics, theology, critical theory and history – to have an interdisciplinary forum for exchanging ideas on how medicine and disease were constructed before cAD1500. *Studies in Early Medicine*, of which this is the first volume, was established as a direct result of the *Disease and Disability* workshops, to address this need.

This new peer-reviewed series is designed to cover the growing discipline of the study of all aspects of disease, disability, health, medicine and society in the ancient and early medieval world, from prehistory to the Middle Ages. *Studies in Early Medicine* is interdisciplinary and multidisciplinary; papers from the fields of anthropology, archaeology, art, history, law, medicine and any other study relating to medicine, health and society in the pre-modern past in any geographical area are welcome.

Volumes will be devoted to a specific theme, interspersed by occasional general volumes, edited by a Guest Editor or Editors by agreement with the General Editors. Some volumes may arise out of conferences and workshops, but submissions of additional papers around the advertised forthcoming themes would be welcomed for consideration. We invite contributions on all aspects of early disease, medicine and healing. Future contributors are kindly asked to consult the associated website: http://disease.nottingham.ac.uk/doku.php.

General Editors

Dr Sally Crawford, Institute of Archaeology, 36 Beaumont Street, Oxford OX1 2PG
sally.crawford@arch.ox.ac.uk

Dr Christina Lee, School of English Studies, University Park, Nottingham NG7 2RD
christina.lee@nottingham.ac.uk

Contents

List of Contributors

Dr Keren Abbou Hershkovits, Institute of Islamic Studies, McGill University, Morrice Hall, 3485 McTavish Street, Montreal, Quebec, Canada.
kabbou@gmail.com

Dr Sally Crawford, The Institute of Archaeology, 36 Beaumont Street, Oxford OX1 2PG, UK.
sally.crawford@arch.ox.ac.uk

Dr Christina Lee, School of English Studies, University Park, Nottingham NG7 2RD, UK.
christina.lee@nottingham.ac.uk

Dr Irina Metzler, Department of History and Classics, Swansea University, Swansea SA2 8PP, UK.
irinametzler@yahoo.co.uk

Dr Anne Irene Riisøy, Institutt for arkeologi, knoservering og historie, University of Oslo, Norway.
Riisøy@iakh.uio.no

Dr Ephraim Shoham-Steiner, Dept. of Jewish History, Ben-Gurion University of the Negev, Beersheba, Israel.
shohamst@bgu.ac.il

Dr Kirsten C. Uszkalo, Department of History, University of Illinois at Urbana-Champaign, Urbana, Illinois, USA.
circe@ufies.org

Chapter One

Introduction

Sally Crawford and Christina Lee

The first scholarly assessments of medieval medicine tended to present the story of medicine as a developing journey from past ignorance to present knowledge, and the practice of medieval medicine has been judged in this context and found wanting.[1] A reaction to this has been to argue that some medieval medicine would have been effective – though recent analyses of early English remedies, for example, have thrown doubt on the arguments of the apologists.[2] To assess the validity of medieval medicine by the efficacy of the remedies is to offer a limited approach to the past, however, and the wider, cultural contexts of medieval medicine have also received increasing attention, alongside a developing awareness that ideas about health and disease, as distinct from biological events affecting the body, are neither natural nor universal features of human groups, but appear as specific structural and cultural components of societies. This is part of looking at medicine not as a simple precursor to modern medical approaches and practices, but as an aspect of social ordering of the world.[3] As a social construct, the definitions of illness in an individual, and individual and group responses to the identification of illness in an individual, are also linked to other variables such as class, age, gender and ethnicity. The social dimension of medical practice was a key theme at the *Disease and Disability in Medieval Europe* workshops, and it is this theme the papers in this first volume of *Studies in Early Medicine* seek to address. Contributors to this volume range from established scholars to new researchers, and contributions include both papers presented at the workshops and additional papers submitted to the editors.

Given that ways of interpreting and responding to illness have a cultural dimension, in many ways illness and its treatment in the past is not well served by being compared to modern medical practice. Rather, interpretations of illness and its treatments can be usefully viewed in a social context, because the categorisation of disease or disability inherently carries assumptions about the nature of the 'well' or 'normal' body and what is 'acceptable' in terms of physical condition may differ from culture to culture.[4] Equally, a society may be understood and interpreted according to the extent to which physical and mental differences are accommodated within the social group, particularly given the permeable and shifting boundaries between 'healthy' and 'unhealthy' according to political, religious and medical developments.[5] The influence of religious belief, whether Christian, Muslim or Jewish, on shaping approaches to health, has been a significant strand in studies of medieval medicine.[6]

The body and its relationship to medicine have been particularly explored in gendered approaches to the past practice of medicine. Women's health and obstetrics have taken a wide room in analyses of medieval medicine and in exploration of the duality of female healers, and medical attitudes towards the female body.[7] Monica Green's recent work on the ways in which the female body and its illnesses were reframed and redefined, with the corollary exclusion of women and control of medical knowledge by men, demonstrates the extent to which medieval medicine, ideas about the body, and acquisition and transmission of medical practice, reflect changes in the framing of medieval society as a whole.[8]

The social complexities of defining a well or healthy body are a recurring theme in the first papers presented in this volume. Disease, especially in a society with little effective medical care, is as much a social and psychological issue as a medical one.[9] This is particularly relevant in the case of mental illness. Mental illness, although now a medical category, was not always so.[10] Mental illness was, and to an arguable extent still is, a social construct, based on social ideas about acceptable and unacceptable social deviance.[11] Even with a modern medical knowledge-base, it is not entirely clear whether mental illnesses fall into the category of diseases (which can be remedied by giving medicine) or of problems of individual socialisation and perception, which might be remedied by counselling and therapy.

Medieval texts, as Kirsten Uszkalo, Anne Irene Riisøy and Irina Metzler show in their contributions, offer us templates about ways of identifying and responding to deviant behaviour in the past. Kirsten Uszkalo's paper highlights the permeability of conceptual categories of madness in her comparison of 'demon possession' in the medieval period with the early modern period. Drawing on a cognitive science approach, she brings new light to the complicated social construct of the identity of the 'possessed' person. 'Rage/demon possession',

[1] Talbot 1967; Bonser 1963; Porter 1997.
[2] Cameron 1993; Riddle 1992; Crawford and Randall 2002; Brennessel, Drout and Gravel 2005.
[3] Lupton 1994, 11-13; Horden 1992; King 2005; Metzler 2006; and see Horden 2009.
[4] Roberts 2000, 51.
[5] Hubert 2000, 3.
[6] Amundsen 1996, 1982.
[7] Green 2008; Rawcliffe 1995; Cadden 1993; Jacquart and Thomasset 1988; Riddle 1992.
[8] Green 2008.
[9] Hubert, 2000, 1-8.
[10] Brooks 2000, 9.
[11] Brooks 2000, 9.

once identified, marked the sufferer as 'other', and this example highlights the acute impact of diagnosis on social identity: illness is unpredictable, and anyone may be afflicted with a sickness at any time.[12] Furthermore, there may be no question of choice – nor any sure way of avoiding becoming 'other' through illness. Uzkalo also raises the issue of the agency of the sufferer in the creation and definition of disease, and equally reminds us through her exploration of demon possession that, in the case of this illness in particular, the presence of an 'audience' to respond to the display of the disease was, in effect, a symptom: illnesses transcend the bodies of the individual and extend to encompass carers and witnesses.

Interesting recent work has focussed on the culpability of the mentally ill: did illness have an impact on legal responsibility, as gender and age did? Was illness an impediment to full citizenship?[13] Whether a sickness is categorized as socially benign and tolerable, or 'dangerous', may fluctuate and depend heavily on circumstances, both personal (age, gender, status) and social. Certain types of illness and disability, recognised socially as marking out deviancy, may also be deliberately manipulated and used to marginalize, punish and exclude. Anne Irene Riisøy's paper shows that, what in other contexts might be seen as 'rage possession' and be treated through medical or religious intervention, in the context of medieval Icelandic society was a condition with important legal and social ramifications. Her paper emphasises the extent to which a determination of 'other' through physical or mental difference could lead to social differentiation or social exclusion. This form of social exclusion on the basis of perceived 'difference' was unlike, for example, religious or ethnic exclusion because it was not a group, but an individual, who was excluded. In the case of Icelandic society, exclusion was on the grounds that the violence of the individual's behaviour deviated from the acceptable codes for violence in a violent society. Perhaps a mad person, as George Orwell perceptively noted, might be defined as being a minority of one.[14]

In order to understand who was in need of medical aid, we need to understand what constituted 'disease' in the past. Studies of medieval medicine interact with contemporary theories of the body and concepts of 'health', as well as perceived deviations from it. Impairment (the physical aspect) is not synonymous with disability (which includes social exclusion).[15] In her paper for this volume, Irina Metzler considers the ways in which legal and medical approaches to the body intersected, this time through the problem of the hermaphrodite. Medieval discussions of the hermaphrodite accentuated the debates between physicians and lawyers over the right to classify the 'normal' body. Hermaphroditism, clear deviancy from the medical model of 'normal', offered (and still offers) a social challenge within a medical construct: is 'health' to be equated with 'functioning' – is a physically 'different' person (who has not got a disease or illness) healthy?[16] Medicine is, in its very nature, about boundaries. Healthy people are not an object of medical attention: it is only when normal health becomes 'abnormal' that it becomes unhealthy, when people move from the normative – in behaviour, appearance, or emotional or physical well being – to the boundaries.

Riisøy, Uzkalo and Metzler all reinforce the evidence that the practice of medicine was not discrete, nor were medical definitions of illness privileged in social interpretations of human behaviour. Riisøy and Uzkalo both discuss aspects of madness, where the relationship between society and the individual negotiated through public performances of witnessing and responding to non-normative behaviour, and where the extent of the sufferer's agency is a key to determining whether definitions of the behaviour – as criminal, possessed, or sick – are determined and defined through legal, ecclesiastical and communal responses, rather than through medicine.

Metzler, Riisøy and Uskalo discuss conditions that challenge society's definitions, and were the source of repeated negotiations and interpretations – sufferers were on the boundaries of definitions, and even, in the case of Metzler's hermaphrodites, challenged medical and theological certainties about knowledge. In her paper, Metzler also argues that disease is about perception – neither disability nor hermaphroditism are illnesses in any modern conventional sense, yet in neither case does the body conform to 'normality'. Both Riisøy's vargs and Metzler's hermaphrodites pose a serious challenge to social definitions of the essence of human identity and personhood.

For the medieval period, 'the meaning of health ...was never confined simply to the health of the body. Medical men and women lived in a world of two lives, this and the next, and two deaths, the death of the body and the death of the soul'.[17] Thus, if body and soul are intrinsically linked, it makes good sense for the church to offer care for both. Such cultural interpretations may even translate into observable differences in the treatment of the body in legal affairs (the integrity of the body is an important aspect of ordeals), or even how it is buried after death. There are differences in the burials of the physically impaired, for example, although we do not completely understand the patterns yet, as recent explorations of this subject in archaeological and documentary contexts for early medieval England have discussed.[18]

The 'superstitious' nature of medieval medicine has drawn considerable attention in surveys of medical practice in the past.[19] While it is important to understand the extent to which medieval medicine was effective, there also needs to be a discussion of the social context in which medicine was practiced and the genre of medical writing.[20] Medical books were more than a method of passing knowledge. The giving of medical books could be an act of prestige and display, and the medical 'value' of the book might lie not just with the written word, but also with the images within books (and images of healing replicated elsewhere), as protection, or aspects of piety and superstition.[21] Sally Crawford, Ephraim Shoham-Steiner

[12] Hubert 2000, 4.
[13] Crawford 2010; Hadley 2010; Turner forthcoming.
[14] Orwell 1948, 83.
[15] Metzler 2006.
[16] King 2005, 5.
[17] Paxton 1992, 92.
[18] Crawford 2010; Hadley 2010; Lee 2008; Reynolds 2009.
[19] Eg Bonser 1963; Grattan and Singer 1976.
[20] Brennessel, Drout and Gravel 2005.
[21] Murray Jones 2006, 22.

and Keren Abbou Hershkovits discuss the broader implications of the act of writing medicine in their papers, looking at the social meanings of medical texts, and what Murray Jones calls 'a broader concept of the rhetoric of healing and medicine in the Middle Ages'.[22]

In her paper, Sally Crawford attempts to place a reading of Old English medical texts in the wider framework of Anglo-Saxon society as it changed from pagan to Christian. She argues that medical texts were not only written as practical medical handbooks for doctors, but their assimilation of information from a wide range of sources means they also conform to an Anglo-Saxon pattern of knowledge acquisition and transmission through texts in a religious framework. Crawford argues that, for the Anglo-Saxons, the amalgamation of folk, Classical and religious elements found in Anglo-Saxon medical texts, far from representing a breakdown of knowledge and rational thinking, was mirrored in a range of contemporary collections of writing, from law codes to poetry. Old English medical compilations may be understood within the broader pattern of Anglo-Saxon perceptions of texts as a medium for accessing and articulating a divinely formed universe through the collection and collation of all forms of knowledge, of which medicine formed only one part.

Anglo-Saxon England lay towards the geographical limits of western medieval society. The focus of Ephraim Shoham-Steiner's paper is another liminal group, this time isolated through their ethnicity. Medieval European Jewish society is noted for its high percentage of literate individuals, but they were, as Shoham-Steiner notes, often obliged, through circumstance, to keep only essential books and texts. In Jewish society, as in other medieval cultures, knowledge transmission through memorization and recitation, without the intermediary of texts, was the norm. In these circumstances, what was committed to writing needs to be given special attention. The act of writing involved a cost and a decision. When medical knowledge was written down, choices were made to fix and transmit ideas through the rare media of ink, hide and scribe. These were not decisions to be taken lightly, and, as both Crawford and Shoham-Steiner demonstrate in their papers, the writing of medicine had to be negotiated within – or, in the case of Jewish texts, literally between - theological imperatives. Similarly, Shoham-Steiner argues persuasively for the need to read Jewish medical marginalia within the wider construct of a society separate from, but operating within, alien cultures, where knowledge and knowledge transfer offered access to status and the potential for economic security in a cultural context where both safety and status were always threatened. Knowledge was a dangerous weapon, though – that which could bring rewards could also be used to discredit and endanger.

Medieval medicine has deep roots in classical medicine and ranges far beyond the European continent. Keren Abbou Hershkovits's paper takes us into the Muslim medieval world, and picks up the themes of the contexts in which medicine was written down. Here, too, knowledge was dangerous, and medical knowledge - particularly knowledge derived from the ethnic and religious 'other' - had to be recast and reinterpreted to conform to appropriate contexts in which it became acceptable. Just as the first papers in this volume assess the ways in which the physical or mental 'other' was either reconfigured to be tolerable, or categorized as 'other', so bodies of knowledge in medieval England, European Jewish and medieval Muslim societies had to be categorized and framed to conform with ideologically-determined norms.

The medical and physical boundaries of the medieval world abound in this volume. Medicine is literally marginal in the case of Shoham-Steiner's paper, it is 'other' for Abbou Hershkovits's Muslims and needed to be assimilated, and it was gathered together with apparently diverse material – including folk medicine and 'pagan' charms – in Anglo-Saxon texts in conformity with collections of knowledge of the day. Bodies were also liminal or marginal - physically, in the case of Riisøy's murdering monsters, physically placed, in their executions and burials, at the margins of society, and at the margins of land and sea, and conceptually, in the case of Metzler's hermaphrodites and Uszkalo's victims (or actors) in 'rage possession'.

Bibliography

Amundsen, D. 1982. 'Medicine and faith in early Christianity' *Bulletin of the History of Medicine*, **56**, 326-50.

Amundsen, D. 1996. *Medicine, Society, and Faith in the Ancient and Medieval Worlds*, London: Johns Hopkins University Press.

Bonser, W. 1963. *The medical background of Anglo-Saxon England: a study in history, psychology, and folklore*, London: Wellcome Historical Medical Library.

Brennessel, B., Drout, M. and Gravel, R. 2005. 'A reassessment of the efficacy of Anglo-Saxon medicine', *Anglo-Saxon England* **34**, 183-195.

Brooks, R. 2000 'Official madness: a cross-cultural study of involuntary and civil confinement based on 'mental illness'' ,in *Madness, disability and social exclusion: the archaeology and anthropology of 'difference'*, World Archaeology **40**, 9-28.

Cadden, J. 1993. *Meanings of Sex Difference in the Middle Ages: Medicine, Science, and Culture*, Cambridge: Cambridge University Press.

Cameron, M.L. 1993. *Anglo-Saxon Medicine*, Cambridge: Cambridge University Press.

Crawford, S. and Randall, A. 2002 'Archaeology and documentary sources; two approaches to Anglo-Saxon medicine', in R. Arnott (ed.), *The Archaeology of Medicine: Papers given at a session of the annual conference of the Theoretical Archaeology Group held at the University of Birmingham on 20 December 1998*, 101-104, B.A.R. International Series 1046, Oxford: BAR Publishing.

Crawford, S. 2010. 'Differentiation in the Later Anglo-Saxon burial ritual on the basis of mental or physical impairment: a documentary perspective', in J. L. Buckberry and A. K. Cherryson (eds.), *Later Anglo-Saxon Burial, c.650 to*

[22] Murray Jones 2006, 24.

1100AD, 91-100, Oxford: Oxbow.

Green, Monica. 2008. *Making Women's Medicine Masculine*, Oxford: Oxford University Press.

Hadley, D. 2010. 'Burying the socially and physically distinctive in Later Anglo-Saxon England', in J. L. Buckberry and A. K. Cherryson (eds.), *Later Anglo-Saxon Burial, c.650 to 1100AD*. Oxford: Oxbow.

Grattan, J.H.G. and Singer, C.J. 1952. *Anglo-Saxon magic and medicine*, Oxford: Oxford University Press.

Horden, P. 1992. 'Disease, dragons, and saints: the management of epidemics in the Dark Ages', in T. Ranger and P. Slack (eds), *Epidemics and Ideas: Essays on the Historical Perception of Pestilence*, 45-76, Cambridge: Cambridge University Press.

Horden, P. 2009. 'What's wrong with early medieval medicine?' *Social History of Medicine*, Advance Access published online on November 3, 2009: Social History of Medicine, doi:10.1093/shm/hkp052.

Hubert, J. 2000. 'Introduction: the complexity of boundedness and exclusion', *World Archaeology* **40**, 1-8.

Jacquart, D. and Thomasset, C. 1988. *Sexuality and Medicine in the Middle Ages*, Trans. Matthew Adamson. Princeton: Princeton University Press.

King, H. 2005. 'Introduction – what is health?' in H. King, (ed), *Health in Antiquity*, 1-11, London: Routledge.

Lee, C. 2008 'Forever young: child burial in Anglo-Saxon England', in S. Lewis- Simpson (ed) *Youth and Age in the Medieval North*, 17-36, Leiden: Brill.

Lupton, D. 1994. *Medicine as Culture: Illness, Disease, and the Body in Western Societies*, London: Sage.

Metzler, I. 2006. *Disability in Medieval Europe: thinking about physical impairment in the high Middle Ages c1100-1400*, London: Routledge.

Murray Jones, P. 2006. 'Image, word and medicine in the Middle Ages', in J. Givens, K. Reeds and A. Touwaide (eds), *Visualizing medieval medicine and natural history, 1200-1550*, 1-24. AVISTA Studies in the History of Medieval Technology, Science and Art, Aldershot: Ashgate.

Orwell, G. 1948. *Nineteen eighty-four*, London: Penguin.

Paxton, Frederick S. 1992. 'Anointing the sick and the dying in Christian Antiquity and the Early Medieval West', in Cambell, S., Hall, B. and Klausner, D. (eds.), *Health, Disease, and Healing in Medieval Culture*, New York: St. Martin's.

Porter, R. 1997. *The greatest benefit to mankind: a medical history of humanity from antiquity to the present*, London: Harper Collins.

Rawcliffe, C. 1995. *Medicine and Society in Later Medieval England*, Stroud: Allan Sutton.

Reynolds, A. 2009. *Anglo-Saxon deviant burial customs*, Oxford: Oxford University Press.

Riddle, J. M. 1992. *Contraception and Abortion from the Ancient World to the Renaissance*, Cambridge: Harvard University Press.

Roberts, C. 2000. 'Did they take sugar? The use of skeletal evidence in the study of disability in past', *World Archaeology* **40**, 46-59.

Talbot, C.H. 1967. *Medicine in Medieval England*, London: Oldbourne.

Turner, W. Forthcoming. 'Town and Country: a comparison of the treatment of the mentally disabled in Late Medieval English Common Law and Chartered Boroughs', in W. Turner (ed) *Medieval Madness and the Law*. Leiden: Brill.

Chapter Two

Rage Possession: A Cognitive Science Approach to Early English Demon Possession

Kirsten C. Uszkalo

Introduction

'Demon possession' is a fluid and dynamic social construct, a conceptual category vested with meaning by members of a given community. As a system with overlapping cultural, religious, and biological underpinnings, demon possession has often resisted exhaustive attempts at satisfactory categorization. The seemingly primal explosions of emotion and extremes of uncharacteristic behaviour, manifest in powerful and dramatic rituals in which demons are confronted and sometimes expelled, cannot be easily reduced to explanatory models that favour medical, historical, anthropological, psychoanalytical, or theological approaches to the exclusion of all others. Recent studies within cognitive science can advance the dialogue productively by suggesting an explanatory model for understanding the role of embodied emotion in giving rise to, and responding to, the external cultural codes of demon possession as they have been internalized individually. In this paper, certain preliminary contours of such a model will be sketched.

While possession constructs shifted significantly over the course of the Middle Ages and through the Early Modern period, both in outward form and in cultural meaning, a unifying thread throughout this evolution is the important and resilient subset of possession behaviours characterized here as 'rage possession'. What follows will focus specifically on two critical periods of this transition: Anglo-Saxon England (the formative period of English Christianity) and Early Modern England (the period of the most prolific and vigorous textual debate about the reality and nature of possession).

Alongside the range of other trance states and physiological disorders with which demon possession has been associated, and alongside periodic expressions of melancholy, anxiety, fear, and grief, one of the more consistent expressions of demon possession in the Western Christian tradition is the powerful display of rage. Swearing, cursing, and raging against God, often accompanied by frightening facial contortions, extreme gestures, uncharacteristic ejaculations, and wild physical violence, all bespoke a foreign entity having displaced the subject's personality. Although in their extremity, these verbal and physical displays invited spiritual or medical explanations, rage, like all affective states, is based, at least in part, on physiological and cognitive constructs. Rage/anger is theorized to be one of the core affective comportments, which include seeking/expectancy, fear, nurturance/sexuality, social bonding/separation distress, and play/joy.[1] This physiological and cognitive grounding for emotions reveals the experience of rage, and, by virtue, rage possession, to be an intimately embodied experience, as opposed to one that necessarily separates the subject from their sense of self. In understanding possession as embodied, we can re-situate the lived experience of possession within the normative human body, making more immediate our understanding of medieval and Early Modern possessions by illustrating how close they may have been to our own cognitive and physiological understanding of anger. Likewise, we can begin to illuminate the differences in the affective displays of possession across a temporal and cultural divide by situating the performance of possession not just within a Christian understanding of demon behaviours and exorcism or dispossession rituals, but also within the social and cultural contexts in which rage was provoked and enacted.[2]

Previous approaches to unpacking possession

The New Testament - the paradigmatic foundation for most subsequent constructs of demon possession in the Christian West - itself reflects a broad understanding of demonic agency, which includes fevers and seizure disorders alongside displacement possession (in which no trace of the host's agency appears to remain).[3] The understanding of possession in the Western tradition was also informed significantly by Antique medical constructs. Although *melancholia* in classical medicine comprised a wide range of states that included both manic and depressive behaviours, by the early centuries AD it was associated principally with depression.[4] In the early Middle Ages, this conceptualization of melancholy does not seem to appear among the conditions for which people were brought to healing shrines or to saints' tombs for healing, or to have been demonized as a condition requiring exorcism. The sin of *acedia*, or 'spiritual sloth', was often described using the rhetoric of demonic instigation and possession, but since it was very narrowly contextualized within monastic disciplines, this has been largely distinguished from broader processes of clinical depression.[5] Isidore of Seville offers a three-fold division of chronic brain disorders, each corresponding to one of the brain's three regions: epilepsy afflicts the frontal region

[1] Thompson 2001, 5.

[2] Discussion of the full role of social neuroscience in the construction of rage possession lies outside the parameters of this essay, but its importance will be suggested throughout.

[3] On displacement possession, from a social cognitive perspective, see Cohen and Barrett 2008, esp. 247 for displacement possession.

[4] Kemp 1989, 73; Toohey 2004, 33-42, 126-27, 154-56. Still useful is Jackson 1986.

[5] On early semantic distinctions in acedia, and the limits of identifying that term with modern clinical depression, see Crislip 2005. For a phenomenological and historical meditation on acedia, see Toohey 2004, 132-57.

(the imagination), melancholy the middle region (reason), and mania the posterior region (memory). Isidore does not say much about melancholy (the same is true of Caelius Aurelianus, one of the conveyers of classical medicine to the Latin Middle Ages), or even mania, but lingers especially on epilepsy. This is the disorder, according to Isidore, especially associated with demonic spirits: *Hos etiam vulgus lunaticos vocant, quod per lunae cursum comitetur eos insidia daemonum. Item et larvatici* ('The common people also call these [epileptics] "lunatics", because the snares of demons accompany them following the course of the moon. Also, "spirit-possessed"').[6] Bede also associates 'lunacy' with demonic influence: *Lunatici dicuntur quorum dolor in ascensione lunae crescebat, non quod inde vere fieret, sed ob daemonum fallaciam...* ('They are called "lunatics" in whom a pain would arise at the rising of the moon, not because it actually originates from that, but through the deceit of demons...').[7] By *lunaticus* or *monaðseoc* ('lunatic', 'month-sick') early commentators may not necessarily have had in mind conditions synchronized with the lunar calendar, but may be referring more loosely to fits or seizures recurring periodically or sporadically.[8] Several Anglo-Saxon cases of possession are evidently epileptic or other seizure disorders: for instance, in Bede's *Ecclesiastical History*, a visitor to Bardney Abbey, *subito a diabolo arreptus clamare, dentibus frendere, spumare et diuersis motibus coepit membra torquere* ('was suddenly seized by the devil and began to cry out, gnash his teeth, foam at the mouth, and fling his limbs about').[9] Alongside the surges of raw energy displayed in epileptic fits, violent outbursts were read as demonic: Anglo-Saxons saw the work of demons where there was a perceived surplus of spleen or energy.[10]

Historically, a range of organic disorders have shared conceptual space with demons and demon possession, and have been attributed to sentient agents having entered and taken over the body. Epileptic seizures can involve series of seemingly deliberative, coordinated activities (e.g., following a familiar domestic routine), after which the subject has no memory of the episode. Obsessive-compulsive ticking, and outbursts or rituals associated with Tourette Syndrome, can appear as willed activities: that is, they involve coordinated gestures in the absence of any visible compelling, external force. However, severe forms of such behavioural anomalies are extremely rare. Only the most dramatic cases, from along the full spectrum, would be potentially threatening to the subject's well being or to the community's sense of stability. While some physiological dysfunctions would have been considered demon possession, other diagnoses were available: even in the Middle Ages, humoral balance and other medical models were applied, albeit inconsistently. How a given case was perceived and treated would have depended on the subjective assessment of caregivers and community, from the family to the available healer or priest.

The vast majority of cases encountered in historical sources - and what is still observable today - are not misunderstood physiological dysfunction, however, but can be thought of rather as 'functional' possession. In functional possession, the behaviours are elicited in specific social contexts, and unfold ritualistically according to the cultural scripting provided by communal beliefs and the individual's prior experience. This does not mean that the subject is conscious of this scripting, or that the behaviours are deliberately invoked or faked in any way (although these possibilities are also documented). Rather, in most cases, they emerge organically as part of an emotionally and religiously charged communal experience. It is important to keep the physiological disorders in mind as part of the historical spectrum, however, because they serve as a cultural model for many of the behaviours in functional possession (e.g., falling to the ground, frothing at the mouth, contorting limbs).

Histories and theologies of possession have been interpretive battlegrounds almost since the earliest appearances of the phenomenon itself in the Western tradition.[11] Christian apologists in the first few centuries AD pointed to possession as proof positive of the correctness of Christianity over local paganisms.[12] In the early Middle Ages, exorcisms were among the most dramatic of healing miracles associated with saints, in an era before the centralized control over the process of canonization and during which the liturgy was heterogeneous and rapidly evolving. In the central Middle Ages, new legal, philosophical, and theological models generated rigorous academic demonology, determining the vocabulary and theoretical problems surrounding possession until well into the Early Modern period.[13] Recent scholars have been interested in gendered aspects of the intertwining of the divine and the demonic in the late Middle Ages and Early Modern periods: debates over whether or not any given visionary was being inspired by God or a demon became a key site of control over local authority.[14] In conjunction with contemporary physiological models that presented fluids and empty spaces as functioning differently in male and female bodies, the ways in which demons can insinuate themselves into the human body was a problem—at the cusp of the era of witch trials—with paramount consequences.[15] In the Reformation, theological debates between Catholicism and Protestant Churches might manifest as competing arguments over the efficacy of exorcism *versus* dispossession. By this period, demon possession had become linked with witchcraft in Western Europe, as the need for a human agent in summoning demonic powers had gained general acceptance. Throughout the 17th and 18th centuries, with the emergence of modern disciplinary categories and methodologies, and with the continued growth of a unified and robust medical discourse, demon possession retreated to the provenance of theology: a respected and rarefied discipline in

[6] Isidore of Seville, *Etymologiarum libri* (Hereafter *EL*) *XX*, 4.7.
[7] Bede, *In Matthaei Evangelium Expositio* 1.4 (*PL* 92, col. 23C).
[8] Temkin 1945, 93.
[9] Bede, *Historia Ecclesiastica (H.E.)* 3.11.
[10] *Energumen*, a common medieval term for 'demoniac', recalls the Greek root *en-ergon* (to work upon) which also gives us 'energy'. *Energuminus* is most commonly glossed in Old English as *gewitseoc* (wit-sick) and *deofulseoc* (devil-sick).

[11] I would like to thank Dr. Peter Dendle of Pennsylvania State University, Mont Alto for collaborating with me on this summary overview of demon possession in the Western tradition, and for his very thorough consultation relating to the Anglo-Saxon period.
[12] E.g., Justin Martyr, *Dialogue with Trypho*, chs. 30, 76, and *1 Apology* 18; Irenaeus, *Against Heresies* 2.32.4; Origen, *Contra Celsum* 7.4.
[13] Boureau 2006.
[14] Caciola 2003; Newman 1998.
[15] Caciola 2005, 21-37.

itself, but one increasingly marginalized from the experimental sciences. In the 19th century, spiritual mediums claimed to channel the deceased and other spirits, even as mainstream Anglican authorities avoided the topic of possession as something of an antiquated superstition.[16] Victorian scholars treated possession mostly as an anthropological curiosity to be studied in remote regions. In the 20th century, psychological and anthropological approaches predominated in the academic study of demon possession: possession behaviour was seen as manifesting psychological impulses in the individual, or social pressures within the community.

The growth of systematic anthropology in the 19th and 20th centuries sparked serious study of various possession paradigms around the world.[17] Structural schools of thought looked for underlying similarities in symptoms and cultural contexts, focusing more on basic patterns of rite, myth, and narrative than on particular circumstances or individual iterations.[18] A growth in available ethnographic data enriched existing paradigms with variant cultural forms of possession and trance states in Haiti and the Caribbean, Sri Lanka, and other places.[19] As these anthropological surveys grew more nuanced and reached a broader readership, demon possession as a matrix of cultural symbols began to intersect - and sometimes jar - with the clinical treatment of schizophrenia and mental disorder in modern therapeutic contexts.[20] In sociology, power relations schools saw in trances and possession behaviours implicit struggles for authority, e.g., women or other marginalized sectors expressed resistance through socially sanctioned channels: 'exorcisms orchestrate a highly disciplined, hieratic message of authority and subordination, which they both enact and explain'.[21] Recent scholarship on possession tends to incorporate elements of sociology, psychoanalysis, and anthropology to various extents, and - sensitive to the fragile particularities of such an adaptive set of beliefs and behaviours - are careful to situate possession narrowly in the unique cultural characteristics of the society in question.[22]

However, psychoanalytical models, pioneered by Sigmund Freud but promulgated in a wide range of schools over the 20th century, proved especially resilient as explanatory tools for the apparent fracturing of self and the extremes of behaviour in the individual.[23] Pubescent subjects suddenly engaging in graphic sexual language or gestures, blaspheming against God, and swearing against loved family and friends, could be read as venting libidinal impulses, frustrated desires, or repressed aggression. In the first half of the 20th century especially, the unconscious was allowed a principal role in a wide range of disorders, implicitly or explicitly considered psychogenic (primarily of mental or emotional origin). Freud's unconscious became, according to Otto Rank, 'a kind of private hell which housed the evil self'.[24] The id was a Pandora's box of passion and aggression, of blind, senseless violence, and of self-destructive potentiality, to be constantly monitored with vigilance, but which could never be completely contained. The object-relations school of thought - to mention but one school built on psychoanalytic axioms - accounted for constructs such as ghosts or demons as projections of the infant's pre-rational perceptions of frustrated desires or aggressive impulses, vestigially perpetuated in mythologized forms into childhood, adolescence, and even adulthood.[25]

In sermon literature, Bible commentary, and other historical interpretations of Christian texts, an implicit hermeneutic not unlike Freud's developed within the discourse of personal spiritual vigilance. The rhetoric of Christian pastoral and devotional literature refers traditionally to demons which invade the mind and body. These are seen as progenitors of all manner of evil impulses, even in the darkest corners of the remotest interiors of the self, to be watched over, warded against, and expelled. The abstract concept of demons, injecting impure thoughts and desires from either inside or outside the human body, allows religious literature to lend itself easily to a modernized lens of psychological impulse. It is no coincidence that modern devotional writers such as Thomas Merton have turned to the ancient Desert Fathers of the first few centuries AD for inspiration and guidance.

This approach suggests something rather the opposite of psychoanalytic models of possession, in which repressed emotional desires and impulses are conceived as building up gradually over time, leading periodically to pitched moments of venting. By that account, the release provided by exorcism or dispossession is thought to relieve the subject in some sense, thus proving a genuinely effective (if not permanent) therapy. One would expect, on a psychoanalytic account, these outbursts to decrease in intensity, in proportion with their frequency. One would also expect an equilibrium to be possible, in which the regular venting of emotion could reach a stable level, predictable and sustainable within the local mechanisms of ritual expression (as is the case in many societies that include trance states as part of regular rituals). This does not seem to accurately reflect numerous descriptions of demon possession in England, either in the Early Middle Ages or the Early Modern period. In the case studies here discussed, such emotional states are exacerbated, each building from prior experiences. Possession behaviour is not symptomatic of an inherent impulse seeking release, but represents a learned affective display that can mutate and intensify over time. In understanding the ways in which the mind and body store emotional states, we can begin to gain better insight into the lived experiences of possession. Linking together some current models of cognitive theory might suggest a preliminary interpretive model for a fuller understanding of the linguistic, cognitive, and physical manifestation of early examples of rage possession.

[16] See comments by Robert Mortimer, Bishop of Exeter, in Petitpierre 1972, 15-16.
[17] An early and influential treatment - outside of more holistic studies such as Sir James Frazer's *The Golden Bough* - is Oesterreich 1930, far more methodologically sound than earlier surveys such as Conway 1881.
[18] E.g., Lewis 1971 and Lewis 1970.
[19] For Haiti and the Caribbean, see Bourguignon 1976; Deren 1953; and Hurston 1938. Gananath Obeyesekere is the researcher most associated with Sri Lanka, with studies such as Obeyeskere 1981 and 1984.
[20] Ferracuti *et al.* 1996; Goff *et al.* 1991; Hale and Pinninti 1994; Leavitt1993.
[21] Caciola 2003, 267. See also Ward 1989, and for use by women as an 'oblique' strategy of resistance, see Chajes 2001, 389.
[22] E.g., Boddy 1989; Dwyer 2003; Greenfield 2008; Keller 2002; Sengers 2003.
[23] See Freud's classic discussion of the topic (1923). For select applications, see Asch 1985; Henderson 1982; and Taylor 1978.
[24] Rank 1958, 38.
[25] Henderson 1982 and Taylor 1978, 53-60. See also Asch 1985, 158-62.

Cognitive and Physiological Embodiments of Rage

Developments in cognitive science have encouraged a return to underlying normative processes as the basis for a study of many aspects of human behaviour. Cognitive science is 'the interdisciplinary study of mind and intelligence, embracing philosophy, psychology, artificial intelligence, neuroscience, linguistics, and anthropology'.[26] Although the field embraces a wide variety of approaches and methodologies, this section will look specifically at the role of language and perceptual symbols as working together to create embodied conceptual understandings that may operate in rage possessions. In *The Embodiment of Emotion*, Lisa Feldman Barrett and Kristen A. Lindquist describe the role of the body in mediating how conceptual systems are formed in response to the individual's own lived experiences. They argue that categories of emotion such as anger and fear are 'instantiated as modality-specific sensorimotor (rather than abstract propositional) representations of prior events, called perceptual symbols'.[27] The location of comprehension within this experiential framework is called 'the perceptual symbols system'. Barrett and Lindquist explain:

> 'neurons in different modalities (e.g., vision, audition, interoception, motor behaviour) capture different sensory and motor elements of a perceptual event, and neural representations accumulate to produce a 'simulator' that serves as a toolbox for creating any future conceptual representation of a category. For example, a simulator for a category of knowledge, like anger, will develop as sensory, motor, and somatovisceral features that are integrated across contexts and settings where instances of anger are labelled... As instances of anger accumulate, and information is integrated across instances, a simulator for anger develops and conceptual knowledge about anger accrues. The resulting conceptual system is a distributed collection of modality-specific memories captured across all instances of a category. These establish the conceptual content for the basic-level category anger, and can be retrieved for later simulations of anger'.[28]

Emotional states are therefore not spontaneous behaviours arising inherently and involuntarily, but are stored and called forth from previous bodily experiences of that state. The body learns and remembers rage, drawing from past physiological expressions. Emotional experiences can thus become richer, more complicated, and more intense over time. The performance of these emotions draws from and reinforces learned behaviours. Moreover, based on multiple physiological experiences (experienced across nerves, muscles, and sensory systems), subjects create conceptual categories. Rage possession draws from these conceptual categories as tools to build the personal, social, and spiritual experience and performance of possession.

Lera Boroditsky and Jesse Prinz argue that although two strains of cognitive science characterize thoughts as composed of perceptual symbols or language-like symbols, a combination of these two elements is 'important in mature human thought'.[29] The alignment of the verbalization and performance of possession could be best understood through a theoretical framework which intersects language, as helping to create the conceptual and emotional understanding of rage, and how, as a perceptual symbol, it is experienced across different bodily systems. Whereas perceptual symbols are built from previous experience as felt and recorded across the body, the addition of language in creating conceptual meaning allows us, according to Lawrence W. Barsalou, to represent abstract concepts across time, perform introspection and metacognition, and better coordinate with other people, allowing more complex social meaning and organization.[30] Previous understandings of the connections between language and bodily experience would be linguistically invoked, and the repetition of emotionally charged phrases could amplify this physical experience during possessions.

The language of pain and rage which appears in these possession accounts was used as a means of heightening narrative tension: it is simply good story telling. However, it also operates to give the reader some indication of the torments the demoniacs were facing. Language represents a cognitive matrix into which various physical and emotional understandings of anger intersect.[31] There is an essential connection between language and action; as Arthur M. Glenberg argues, 'cognition is for action'.[32] Recent studies have tracked the interconnection between language and action, suggesting that parts of the body associated with mobility are unconsciously initiated in reading accounts of action. Mentally processing narratives of motion involves mental simulation of that motion: the more strenuous the narrative action, the more time it takes to process it.[33] As such, the comprehension, articulation, and reception of emotive terms can 'activate experiential representations of words (lexical, grammatical, phonological, motoric, tactile) as well as associated experiential representations, and often combinations of these'.[34] The languages of shattering pain and sustained suffering may have given readers, as they would have given the communities which gathered around the demoniac, some organic sense of the physiology of possession: in seeing and hearing it, they could themselves be unconsciously simulating aspects of possession. Articulations of rage are thereby psychologically and socially problematic, including both verbal (swearing, cursing, and blaspheming) and pre-verbal (growling, shouting, or speaking in tongues). These linguistic signifiers are both experiential and communicative. Gestures, furthermore, can serve as a midpoint between embodiment and language: the same part of the brain, Broca's area, controls the lips, the tongue, and the hand.[35]

Rage possession is linguistically and physiologically experienced, not just by the possessed - though there is

---

26 Zalta 2009.
27 Barrett and Kristen 2008.
28 Barrett and Lindquist 2008, 247.
29 Boroditsky and Prinz 2008, 99.
30 Barsalou 2008.
31 Barrett and Lindquist, p. 253. Also see Lindquist *et al.* 2006.
32 Glenberg 2008.
33 Ibid. 49. Also see McNeill, Duncan, Cassell and Levy 2007, and Matlock 2004, 1389-1400.
34 Zwann 2004, esp. 38.
35 McNeill 1992.

certainly a feedback loop between what the demoniac says and does - but also by those who physically and textually observe the possession. The discovery of mirror neurons (neurons which fire when an action is performed, or an action is seen to be performed),[36] and current work in similar functions of empathy,[37] suggest that seeing emotive facial expressions, or even reading about action, can invoke empathetic reactions and unconscious mimicry. The division between self and others, on this neurological level, is believed to blur, creating empathy which itself facilitates the creation of social networks. The social systems at play within the following case studies speak both to the communal creation and proliferation of possession experiences and to the effect the demoniac's actions, words, and gestures had on that community. The community around them felt the anger of the possessed and mirrored it back. These cognitive science concepts can thus help build a framework in which to situate rage possession, one which recognizes it as encompassing the sinews and the senses of the possessed, as an intensely intimate and necessarily social experience, and one which is as gestural and guttural as it is articulate and complex.

Anglo-Saxon Constructs of Rage Possession

Possession was associated especially with neurological or muscle-control disorders, along with behavioural disturbances, unexplained violence, and sudden or intermittent episodes of anger or aggression.[38] As far as the Anglo-Saxon idiom of possession is recorded in extant saints' lives, medical books, laws, and liturgy, the category was widely deployed to explain unchecked excesses of physical power and animation. Demon possession seems to have come to partially occupy the conceptual space occupied by mania in classical medicine. Words for demon possession and its associated states (e.g., madness, lunacy), for instance, have especially strong connections with rage or fury in the glossaries. The late-10th or early-11th century Harley Glossary contains a range of terms for madness, possession, and rage, implying a clear connection between possession and violence:

> freneticus: demoniaticus, insanus, amens, gewitleasa
> frenesis: insanitas
> funeste: funere pollutus, cruente, insaniente, wedende
> furor...reþnes, wodendream
> furis: insanis, erras, bacharis
> furia: insania, amentia, vel dea wodscipe, reþnes
> furias: insania, vel deas, iras, reþscipas vel hatheortnessa
> furalia (read furiale): seua, reþe
> furiosus: iracunda, rabidus, insanus, amens[39]
>
> [frenetic: demoniac, insane, senseless, witless
> frenesis: insanity
> destructive: polluted with death, blood-thirsty, insane, mad
> fury...savagery, mad ecstasy
> you are raving: you are insane, you stray, you rave wantonly
> fury: insanity, senselessness, or the goddess of raving, rage
> the Furies: insanity, or goddesses, wrath, raging or 'hot-heartedness'
> furious: ferocious, savage
> furious: ireful, enraged, insane, senseless]

Here, classical medical categories (*frenesis*, *furia*) are blended with mythological beings (the Furies: glossed in a hybrid Latin-Old English phrase as *dea wodscipe*, or 'goddess of raving'), and both are mixed with a range of concepts referring to diverse mental aberrations (*gewitleasa*, witless; *insanus*, insane; *wodendream*, mad ecstasy or mad happiness). On balance, these show a pronounced emphasis on states of aggressive fury: e.g., *reþnes* (savagery or ferocity), *hatheortnessa* (hot-heartedness or wildness of spirit), *seua* (ferocious), and *rabidus* (enraged). The mid-10th century gloss in MS British Library, Cotton Cleopatra A.iii (probably produced at Canterbury), furthermore, glosses *furias* (the Furies) with *wuhunga* (rages), and the 11th-century Antwerp Glossary equates *furiis* with *gyde* (crazy, possessed, foolish, dizzy), *malignis spiritibus* (wicked spirit), and *mid awyridum gastum* (with unclean spirits).[40] This is what early medieval observers potentially perceived in the ravings of an angry subject. Furthermore, these lexical referents lean toward active savagery rather than passive madness: words for insanity are coupled with words for violence (e.g., *cruente*, blood-thirsty, blood-stained, cruel). The word cluster is a hybrid of Latin and vernacular, of mythological, medical, and theological, drawing from different language and textual communities.

Representing possession as looking like madness and rage suggests a desire to articulate possession as a linguistic concept and as an embodied emotional state. Among other approaches, Niedenthal *et al.* note that semantic network theories locate emotional knowledge within abstracted amodal concepts, such as feature lists with word-like entries. They argue that an anger feature list might be represented as: 'ANGER [frustration, fists clenched, face red, yelling, cursing]'.[41] This paper frames rage possession as located, as Boroditsky and Prinz suggest, within embodied cognition and language like symbols. Of course, at an obvious level, early medieval glossaries are by their very nature simple word lists, compiled for various purposes. Yet, as integral texts themselves, they implicitly emphasize certain language concepts, and order them in patterns which can then carry unique and potentially meaningful valences. They are not unlike litanies of the saints in this regard, which at

[36] Mirror neurons were discovered in non human primates, but have been theorized to function in a similar fashion in humans. See Keysers and Gazzola 2009; Marco *et al* 2005; Ferrari *et al.* 2003.

[37] Lamm *et al.* 2007. Also see Schulte-Ruther *et al.* 2007.

[38] This assertion is argued in greater detail in Dendle forthcoming. In the early Middle Ages, "demons" or "the demonic" represented a much broader concept than in later periods. Consistent with conceptualizations of illness in many pre-modern cultures worldwide, Anglo-Saxons popularly considered a wide range of mental, physical, and behavioural disorders "demonic" in a fundamental sense. Furthermore, these were not well distinguished from crop blights, storms, invasions, and other misfortunes. For previous attempts at taxonomies of possession or mental disorders in Anglo-Saxon England, see Bonser 1963, 257-58; Meaney 1992; Clarke 1975, 73.

[39] Items in Oliphant 1966.

[40] Cleopatra Glossary: Stryker 1951, 209; Antwerp Glossary: Goossens 1974, 441.

[41] Niedenthal et al. 2009 argue that semantic network models of emotion hold that emotions impose structure on information; emotions and affective states alike anger would be represented by a node which links ideas associated with anger. Experiencing emotions would activate that node, spreading across associated nodes and bringing those ideas to mind. The process can work in reverse – the activation of information in the emotional network can generate the emotion.

one level are simply lists of names, but which implicitly draw out the ineffable holiness, righteousness, and obedience that presumably unite the disparate items. In this light, the feature lists in the above glosses usefully map onto the language-like feature lists of emotional concepts; the glosses can be read as an attempt to articulate semantic network cognition. However, the language used to articulate these concepts has the potential for an embodied response for the writer and reader; Niedenthal *et al.* argue that processing conceptual content, even in the form of reading emotive words, involves some reenactment of the emotional state.[42] The word clusters integrate associations, articulating rage possession as conceptually and physically understood, yet resistant to a clear and exhaustive linguistic definition. These glosses - through the network of interrelated terms - indicate what rage possession was and what it felt like: ferocious, angry, and insane. The following narratives flesh out the explication of rage possession as a concept which language can only partially articulate.

Felix's *Life of Guthlac* (c. 730-740?) provides one of the earliest and most detailed narrative descriptions of demon possession in England. A young East Anglian nobleman named Hwætred is seized unexpectedly by a demon. The sudden onset is contrasted with what Felix specifies is a regular pattern of dutifulness and respect:

> One day when he was sitting at home, a wretched spirit suddenly began to attack him. He was stricken with such intense madness that he lacerated his own limbs with wood, iron, and with his own nails and teeth as much as he could. Not only did he tear at himself cruelly and madly, but he also lacerated anyone he could reach with his teeth. He became so insane that he could not, by any means, be hindered or bound. Once when a large group had gathered around him and some of them tried to bind him, he grabbed a honed, double-edged axe and sent three men to the ground with gleeful blows, killing them.[43]

This new stage of Hwætred's life continues for four years, until the man is all but wasted. Despite his being taken to various holy men for healing, none of them is able to 'extinguish the pestilential slime [or 'poison'] of the deadly spirit' (*pestiferum funesti spiritus virus exstinguere*). The crowding in and periodic attempts at binding presumably fuelled a desperate situation. In an Old English interpretation of this passage, the anonymous Anglo-Saxon translator adds a detail not found in the original: the crowd gathered around him is comprised of his 'family' and 'close friends'.[44] This community's movement toward control and integration only makes the situation worse: these attempts feed the rage, rather than diffuse it. His parents bind and carry Hwætred away from the community which exacerbated his rage possession to the isolated fen island of Crowland, where Guthlac sequesters himself with the man for three days of prayer and fasting. On the third day, Guthlac breathes into the man's face (a ritual action known as *insufflation*), and the man is relieved of his long-standing affliction all at once. His behavioural response is to 'draw long sighs from deep in his heart' (*longa suspiria imo de pectore trahens*). Thus, he answers Guthlac's symbolic breath with a parallel action, but one described in biological rather than ritual terms. Hwætred finds in Guthlac a new mode of behaviour to mimic and with which to synchronize - that of peaceful and ritualized prayer. Exhaustion and emaciation, distance from the environment which reinforced his identity as a demoniac, and intimate physical and psychological proximity to Guthlac, may have created a situation where the boundaries between the two men partially dissolved.[45] Hwætred is never again afflicted by demons after he has temporarily fused his behaviours and his sense of self with Guthlac.

In a letter of c. 746-747 AD co-written with seven other bishops, Boniface praises King Æthelbald of Mercia for giving alms, suppressing crimes, and protecting the widowed and the poor. The tone soon shifts to admonishment, however. Æthelbald has 'not taken a lawful wife' and is 'driven by lust into the sins of fornication and adultery' committing 'these sins, to [his] greater shame, in various monasteries with holy nuns and virgins vowed to God'.[46] As he has violated the brides of Christ, Æthelbald also violated *the* bride of Christ - the churches and monasteries. He has 'filched away their revenues' while allowing his 'governors and earls use greater violence and oppression towards monks and priests than any other Christian kings have ever done before'.[47] Raping nuns, stealing from churches, and abusing clergy is business as usual, Boniface laments. Osred, King of Bernicia and Deira, and Ceolred, King of Mercia, were both tempted by evil spirits to sexually assault nuns and destroy monasteries. However, he is quick to add, both Kings paid for ecclesiastical and sexual violations with their souls. Osred, who 'maddened and spurred on by his lust, outraged consecrated virgins in their convents' lost both 'his life and his soul until a shameful and ignominious death deprived him of his glorious kingdom, his young wife and his impure soul'.[48] Boniface alleges that Ceolred's sins of aggression and exploitations turned inward, and he lost his power, his mind, and his soul:

> as those who were present testify, sat feasting amidst his nobles, an evil spirit which had seduced him into defying the law of God suddenly struck him with madness, so that still in his sins, without repentance or confession, raving mad, gibbering with demons and cursing the priests of God, he departed from this life and went certainly to the torments of hell.[49]

---

[42] *Ibid.* 1113.

[43] 'quadam die domi sedens, subito illum nequam spiritus grassari coepit. In tantum autem inmensa dementia vexabatur ita ut membra sua propria ligno, ferro, unguibus dentibusque, prout potuit, laniaret; non solum enim se ipsum crudeli vesania decerpebat, quin etiam omnes, quoscumque tangere potuisset, inprobi oris morsibus lacerabat. Eo autem modo insanire coepit, ut eum prohiberi aut adligari nullius ausibus inpetraretur. Nam quodam tempore, congregata multitudine, cum alii illum ligare temtarent, arrepto limali bipenne tria virorum corpora letabundis ictibus humo sternens mori coegit'. Felix, *Vita Guthlaci*, ch. 41 (Colgrave 1956, 126-28).

[44] *Maga* and *nehfreonda* (Gonser 1909, 146). The prose vernacular version of the *Life of Guthlac* was probably written in the 9th century, perhaps associated with the literacy campaign of Alfred the Great.

[45] Semin and Cacioppo 2008, 119-147.

[46] Boniface, Letter 73 (Tangl 1955, 152).

[47] *Ibid.*, 153.

[48] *Ibid.*, 153.

[49] 'Nam Ceolredum, precessorem venerande celsitudinis tuae, ut testati sunt qui presentes fuerant, apud comites suos splendide epulantem malignus spiritus, qui eum ad fiduciam dampnandae legis Dei suadendo pellexit, peccantem subito in insaniam mentis convertit, ut sine penitentia et

The anger and aggression Ceolred outwardly indulged in, turned inward: the fury and the raving of the rapist becomes the senseless raving of the demoniac. Theresa A. Gannon lists some social-cognitive perspectives which help to explain aggressive and violent behaviour, including script theory (the normalization and automatic nature of violent responses), cognitive neoassociation (the connection between different aggressive concepts, in this case sexual and political violence), and implicit theories (the normalization of violence as pre-emptive and judgmental).[50] Boniface paints Ceolred as surrounded by compatriots (*comites*), once again situating the ravings of the individual within a community who clearly normalize and reinforce his aggressive behaviour. It is unclear whether 'conversing with devils' is to be visualized as literally engaging invisible spirits in conversation, or perhaps surrounding himself with bad company, or perhaps engaging in impious pursuits and conversation. The physical violation of the nuns and spiritual dissolution of the monasteries lead to Ceolred's own physical and spiritual dissolution.[51] His undue determination to sexually and economically possess and violate the Church lead to Ceolred's own possession and violation. Raging and damned, he dies. Boniface suggests that if Æthelbald continued to normalize aggression, rape, and robbery, as his predecessors did, that he would follow the same route, and become possessed by the power he unrightfully claimed.

These cases are resonant with other medieval cases from the continent, which return periodically to visceral explosions of anger as quintessentially demonic. Demoniacs drop to the ground and pound their fists; they rail and beat themselves with their hands until bloody, possessed by a 'raging demon'. They 'rave wildly' and cry out.[52] A woman in the *Life of Radegund* 'raved so violently that she shook the whole basilica with her roaring'.[53] Another woman in the same passage has been assaulted violently by a demon for fifteen years. A woman in Gregory the Great's *Dialogues* is infested with a legion of demons: 'it seemed that all the devils together were wildly agitating her body, shouting and screaming furiously'.[54] Bodies are described as straining and contorting, tensed and convulsed, held down by onlookers and bound up in chains. Braulio of Saragossa's *Life of Aemilian the Confessor* tells of a certain deacon possessed by a demon: 'he was convulsed by his madness as if he was rabid, raving and lashing out'.[55] Medieval sources are never as detailed as the modern scholar might wish, and hagiography by its very nature adheres to a restricted range of commonly repeated tropes and phrases, but the picture that emerges reveals a consistent association of rage with demon possession, underlying local variation.

Demons operate in these early medieval narratives not as traditional literary devices or monovalent symbols for sin or disease, but as amorphous constructs that shift over time and that operate variously within the same society and often even within the same text. They are abstractions, but abstractions returning time and again to the language of physiology and to the embodied experience of suffering individuals at the heart of a communal nexus. Understanding how these conceptual constructs function sets the stage usefully for the much more fully documented possession behaviours that appear in the Early Modern period.

Early Modern Constructs of Rage Possession

Apart from conjuring a kind of salacious pleasure or *Schadenfreude* within a moralizing textual framework, there appears to be some desire in Early Modern England to align inexplicable anger with the presence of angry foreign entities. James concludes *Daemonologie* (1597) with a warning to his readers, as do a number of contemporary authors, that the approach of the end of days 'makes Satan rage more in his instruments, knowing that his kingdom be so near an end'.[56] Along with the rise in witch prosecutions, prophets, and texts about prodigious wonders, stories of malevolent mothers, ghosts, faeries who physically and emotionally torment witting and unwitting victims are recounted across a variety of later textual sources, including encyclopaedias of supernatural occurrences like Joseph Glanvill's *Sadducismus Triumphatus* (1681), George Sinclair's *Satan's Invisible World Discovered* (1685), and Richard Bernard's *The Certainty of the Worlds of Spirits* (1691). There is a great deal of discursive and definitional slippage in these varied texts: emotions are embodied in malefic malformations which define women as witches; in the monster babies which manifest the moral, spiritual, or political deviancies of their parents; in the prone and starving frame of the ecstatic prophet; and the relentless door knocking of their missionary sibling. All of these bodies were read, at least in part, as providing affective performances, and amidst all the visceral and verbal displays of anxiety and anger, it is often difficult to tease out cases of possession as we would understand them. Possession appears in many different forms. Moshe Sluhovsky distinguishes two distinct forms of early English possession phenomena: one type of possession takes the form of an invasion by a possessing agent resolved by exorcism; the second type, which operates as a malefic disease

confessione furibundus et amens et cum diabolis sermocinans et Dei sacerdotes abhominans de hac luce sine dubio ad tormenta inferni migravit.' *Ibid.*, 153.

[50] Script theory suggests that individuals learn 'aggressive concepts and sequences during childhood that - following excessive rehearsal and strengthening - become chronically accessible, automated behavioural responses'. Cognitive neoassociation is the theory that aggressive concepts and emotions (including behavioural sequences) are linked within long-term memory such that highly related concepts, and those typically activated in unison form strong associative bonds. Implicit Theories suggest that that offenders 'normalised violence (i.e. as a normal and necessary part of existence) providing an important cognitive backdrop to two other implicit theories: beat or be beaten (i.e. beliefs that violence is required in order to attain independence and status within a hostile world) and I am the law (i.e. beliefs that one is entitled to morally judge others' behaviours and administer retribution accordingly)' (Gannon 2009).

[51] Boniface knew it was coming; the Monk at Wenlock saw a vision of the Devils crowding around Ceolred and convincing the disheartened Angels who had protected him Ceolred to give up: he had committed 'a multitude of horrible and unspeakable crimes', and they needed to be let in to mete out retribution (Kylie 1911, 87).

[52] Gregory of Tours: *Life of Julian* (Krusch 1885, 128, 129) and *Life of Martin* (Krusch, 167).

[53] This is found in Baudonivia's supplement to Venantius Fortunatus' *Life of Radegund* (Book 2): ch. 27 (Krusch 1888, 394); trans. McNamara and Halborg 1992, 104.

[54] Gregory the Great, *Dialogi* 1.10: 'Coepit ex hoc illa tot motibus agitari, tot uocibus clamoribusque persrepere, quot spiritibus tenebatur' (de Vogüé 1979, 96; Zimmerman 1959, 43).

[55] Braulio of Saragossa, ch. 12, col. 707D: 'more lymphatico amentia ageretur furens grassatus'; trans. Fear 1997, 29.

[56] Almond 2004, 13-14.

played out in the body of a victim, originates with a demonic contract and terminates with the witch's death.[57] There are instances of verbal and visceral anger which help construct and define both types of possession scenario.

In the case of possession bewitchments, language empowered the speaker and disempowered the listener. Merely enunciating negative words could also set malefic magic in progress. Especially bad language could penetrate listeners, growing, tormenting, and possessing them. Keith Thomas argues for the nebulousness of linguistic signifiers, which contributed to the 'making of a witch'.[58] Scolding, cursing, and blaspheming women commonly appear in witchcraft narratives, tracts, and salacious accounts. Ill-timed or ill-used speech could condemn women. Christina Larner argues that the 'women who went to the stake during the witch-hunt went cursing, often for the crime of cursing'.[59] The person who decided the difference between a curse and a malefic spell also determined if the speaker was a witch.[60] These women were as angry as they sounded. The articulation of rage gave their curses malefic power. Moreover, behind the words lay the spiritual or moral corruption where rage could breed.

Possession by rage was like possession by demons. It created an opportunity for the devil, in one way or another, to possess the cursers. Mary Smith was angry about cheese. Alexander Roberts' *A Treatise of Witchcraft* (1620) recounts the story of how a shop set up by her neighbours threatened Smith's entrepreneurial sale of Holland cheese. Smith was irate and:

> often times cursed them, and became incensed with unruly passions, armed with a settled resolution, to effect some mischieuous proiects and designes against them: attracted the devil in the shape of a Blackman who encouraged her to 'malice, enuy, hatred, banning and cursing' and promising her revenge entered into a contract with her.

The devil wanted to keep Smith angry so as to 'hold her still in his possession'.[61] The correlation of cursing with invoking devils appears in numerous cases. Joan Flower's 'oathes, curses, and imprecations irreligious' made her a 'monstrous malicious woman' and 'a plaine Atheist', continually under suspicion because of the type of language she freely used.[62] Elizabeth Sawyer began her confession by stating that 'the first time that the Devil came unto me was, when I was cursing, swearing, and blaspheming'.[63] She claimed that 'he then rushed in Upon me and never before that time did I see him, or he me: and when he, namely the Divel, came to me, the first words that hee spake unto me were these: Oh! have I now found you cursing, swearing, and blaspheming? now you are mine'. Most famously, Anne Bodenham refused to confess, recant, or even travel to the gallows sober, and declared that she 'had as many prayers already as she intended, and desired to have, but cursed those that detained her from her death, and was importunate to goe up the Ladder'.[64] To the last minute, Bodenham refused to incorporate herself into the standard plot, or deliver the standard lines: when the 'Executioner stayed her, and desired her to forgive him: She replyed, Forgive thee? A pox on thee, turn me off; which were the last words she spake'.

Cognition and motion are linked. The brain processes action and action words in similar ways; the same parts of the brain fire when we read action words as do when we perform those actions. But what happens in terms of the processing of more abstract terms like cursing, swearing, and blaspheming? How does the body process these words which do not necessarily have an accompanying action?[65] Boroditsky and Printz argue that the mind can process abstract concepts within the perceptual symbol system based on the use of conceptual metaphors, scripts (socially appropriate ways of acting), and emotional responses.[66] It is likely that those producing and suffering from curses understood them, at least in part, through these strategies. At the very least, cursing functioned to frighten, and its performance was culturally scripted. Moreover, although the curse could have been seen as an abstract concept, the power malefic languages carried was understood through experience and examples. Cursing was part of what made a woman a witch, but the reported torments and murders associated with maleficium enabled her identification and persecution as one. The accounts we have of cursing women, like the tales of demoniacs, are produced after the fact; the results of the curses are already given a conceptual framework: the devil came and made women witches and the behaviours altered and their bodies changed. The abstract made sense in hindsight. Languages of rage performed by alleged witches therefore served as models for the performance of raging possession by demoniacs - acting as scripts or prompts for linguistic signifiers of embodied experiences. Linguistic and physical displays illustrate a potential slippery slope between early articulations and the eventual experience of rage possession.

Locating the violent actions of demoniacs within this framework allows us to recognize some of their fits and torments as human expressions of anger.[67] Although we might

[57] Sluhovsky 2002, 256.
[58] Thomas 1971, 502.
[59] Larner 2002, 274.
[60] Larner (2002, 273) argues that women had two kinds of linguistic powers derived from the established order: the power to 'defend herself or to curse'. Clark (1997, 282), while arguing for the efficacy of written and spoken word magic, proposes that 'charms, spells, and curses produced physical changes in objects and persons; actions done to images were conveyed to the things the images depicted; talismans drew down harmful qualities from higher powers'. Suggett (2000, 91) traces the 'significant correspondences between witchcraft and cursing' in early modern Wales. He cites Thomas Cooper, who in 1617 illustrated the danger of angry public speech acts by claiming that '"when a bad-tongued woman shall curse a party, and death shall follow shortly, this is a shrewd token she is a witch", even when "invocating upon her bare knees (for so the manner is) the vengeance of God"' (Suggett 2001, 92). On curse tablets, see Apps and Gow 2003, 123-124.
[61] Roberts 1616, 45.
[62] Anon 1619, C2.
[63] Goodcole 1621, C-C1.
[64] Bower 1653, 39, 36.
[65] Collier argues that the debate over whether we understand ideas in terms of abstraction or through examples which raged in early modern philosophy has yet to be sold by cognitive science, which in many ways replays the same argument, advancing, but not concluding it (2005, 197–207).
[66] Boroditsky and Printz 2008, 104.
[67] Not all possession or bewitchment possession cases are associated with rage or rage possession. A noteworthy example is that of Jane Stretton, who was 'taken with violent rageing fits, which torment her greviously' (M.Y. 1669, 4). However, suggestive cases like Stretton's with its raging fits and torments may be indicative of rage possession, and that of famed faster Martha Taylor who is mentioned in the introduction to Stretton's texts, serve a different textual and social function: they are narratively constructed as cases of the prodigious

not know why they fixated on their victims (the witches accused of tormenting them or the ministers appointed to help them), we can understand, in part, how the performance rage was reified. Each fit could provide another experience to reflect on in the stillness of paralysis and to call on in the frenzy of violent fits. The terrible torments outlined in the following cases complicated and compounded as the possession lengthened. Possession experiences would have come to have their own physiological and conceptual weight, allowing the experience to continue beyond that of a rage which would burn out at the limits of human (and even super human) exhaustion. This suggests that experience enriched each iteration of possession; each previous fit provided more cognitive and physiological information to invoke in the next.[68]

The young maid in Mrs. Hopper's *Strange News from Arpington near Bexly in Kent* (1679) 'was possest with several devils or evil spirits' who would 'talk and shriek within her'.[69] Based on their 'unruly and uncompassionate rage' she would suffer violent and dreadful fits in which she would contort her body, draw back her eyes, bare her teeth, and snarl.[70] Once, in a dreadful tone, the demons distinctly exclaimed: 'weaker and weaker, weaker and weaker', frightening all the observers in the room with what may have been an acknowledgement of their own frailty, or the maid's.[71] One of the demons was drawn out of the maid's mouth and, in the shape of a snake, immediately attempted to strangle the physician who was attempting to dispossess her. Even after this, the spirit inside her continued to make hideous murmurings 'as though it dislikes its present habitation'.[72] The postscript ends with the mention of the maid's continuing possession. Although the maid had brief moments where the demons 'sometimes suffered her a little freedom', the duration of her rage possession out-spanned its narrative context, suggesting that there were enough visitors, including the author, 'who come to see, and all return with the same acknowledgement that they had never saw nor heard of the like all their lives'.[73]

The maid's possession could have continued simply because it was popular: she remained possessed as long as people kept coming to see a demoniac. However, its prodigious length suggests an authenticity to the maid's possession. An audience which was providing affective feedback would have kept the rage possession going, and kept the raging demon, albeit reluctantly and angrily, within the maid. The astonished audience may have been unconsciously mimicking the maid's facial expressions back to her, demonstrating their (neurologically hardwired) empathy. In facing her with fear and awe, they unwittingly continued the feedback loop by continuing to look at the maid. Possession, like empathy, is cognitively and physiologically experienced; as such, it can be seen and felt, and perhaps can move across bodies. The demon's discomfort, suffering, and rage play a part in this story. The demon's mistily serpentine shape functions as a lapsarian symbol, suggesting that the demon itself is an embodiment of possession, and by virtue, that possession is embodied. The demon's movement from the maid to the priest speaks to the role of the social in creating, mirroring, and prolonging possessions (the priest participates in prolonging the possession experience through his exorcism efforts) and speaks to the contagious nature of possessions (which can spread through houses and communities). Moreover, rage possession can be caught, not because a single demon becomes legion, but rather because the possession experience is one which is essentially comprehensible, and experienced through the individual and the social body. If one has the fodder to make rage, one has the embodied understanding to live rage possession. The community which feels for the maid could also feel as she did.

Possession came by way of tattling for Christian Shaw. Francis Grant Cullen's *Sadducismus Debellatus* (1696) recounts that her alleged possession began in Renfrew, Scotland, when Shaw reported a maid whom she saw stealing milk.[74] In retribution, the 'Maid (being a young Woman of a proud and revengeful Temper, and much addicted to Cursing, Swearing and Purloining) did, in a mighty Rage, imprecate the Curse of GOD three times upon the Child; and at the same time did thrice utter these horrid words, The Devil harle (that is Drag) your Soul thro' Hell'.[75] Shaw's encounter with 'one Agnes Naismith, an old ignorant Woman, of a Malicious Disposition, addicted to Threatnings, (which sometimes were observed to be followed with fatal Events)', was also read as suspect. Shaw responded rather flippantly to Naismith's polite inquiry about her family: her fits began the day after. The narrative spends a great deal of time in the first forty pages looking at Shaw twisting, contorting, and producing supernatural effluvia associated with bewitchments.[76] Her moods would sometimes change violently and she would fall into 'freting and angry fits, in which she was cross to all those about her, nothing they did or said proving to her satisfaction'.[77] However, the tone changes by the later half of the text. The apothecary, Mr. Henry Marshall, testified that Shaw's ire was a defining element of her possession experience. He noted that on at least two occasions Shaw flew into a fit, which seems to be more argument than torment. At first 'she had lain so for some time, she arose in a great Rage, beat all about her, Frowning with her Countenance, and uttering a great deal of unknown Language in an Angry manner'.[78] Secondly, having failed to come to a consensus in an argument with an invisible tormentor name Ketie, 'immediately she fell into another Fit, and Swoon'd; and out of that into another Rage, wherein she bit her own Fingers,

and miraculous. However, Stretton's case of bewitchment possession contains various behaviors associated with rage possession in the 17th century, including the involvement of a witch as a catalyst, and 'extraordinary and unusual fits, her abstaining from sustenance for the space of 9 months, being haunted by imps or devils' (M.Y. 1669, 3), which appear in a number of British accounts of bewitchment possession.

[68] For a comprehensive list of some of the more famous demon possession cases in England, see Almond 2004. Although there is some crossover with Almond's text, also see Sands 2004 for some lesser known cases.

[69] Hopper 1679, 2.

[70] *Ibid.* 2.

[71] *Ibid.* 3-4.

[72] *Ibid.* 6.

[73] *Ibid.* 6.

[74] Cullen 1698.

[75] Cullen 1698, 1.

[76] Christian Shaw allegedly brought up 'Tufts of Hair, Straw long, and folded together, burnt Coals, pieces of Bones, Leather, Chips of Timber, and several other things' (Cullen 1698, 41). Vomiting pins and other foreign objects signifies a temporary release of the unnatural agents which alleged witches put into their victims to torment them.

[77] Cullen 1698, 14.

[78] *Ibid.* 42.

and tore her Hands upon Pins that were in her Cloathes; after which she appeared Angry, pulled out all the Pins, and threw them away'.[79]

Like many young female demoniacs in Early Modern England, Shaw may have been practicing possession as a power grab. Cursed by witches, excused from familial responsibilities, and free from her role as a good little girl, Shaw was free to receive all of the (negative) attention a person could want. Her actions clearly point to the scripts and perceptual symbols Christian Shaw called on to produce her possession: Shaw only knew a few ways to express her displeasure. She had temper tantrums and fights with other girls; she liked having things her way and did *not* like it when that did not happen. The sustainability and ferocity of her rages when directed outward suggest a dialogic aspect to her possession experience: even without outside interference, Shaw created, in Ketie, an enemy to fight. She was equally angry when she awoke to discover she had painfully bitten and torn her skin with pins, and disarmed herself of the weapons she had on hand. Shaw's rage was not directional, but fluid and indiscriminate. Gerhard Stemmler notes that emotions function in part to 'allocate perceptual, cognitive, and bodily resources to accomplish the emotion's goals'.[80] Shaw's rage seemed to exist to satisfy itself. Only in trying to satisfy or sate her did the community around Shaw create a focus for her possession: themselves. This narrative, as many narratives about possessions do, seeks to name and understand an experience which is outside explanation. For Shaw it was enough that it was experienced.

Richard Dugdale sold his soul to the devil to become a good dancer. Thomas Jollie, in *The Surey Demoniack* (1697), emphasized how the 'strange fits which violently seized' Richard Dugdale made him 'rage as if he has been nothing but a devil in Richard's bodily shape' for months on end.[81] Dugdale would get himself drunk and be 'transported into such a state of profaneness that as did astonish bystanders'.[82] Beyond displaying bad temper and violence, which could also be associated with long nights of dancing and drinking, Dugdale also displayed bizarre contortions, rolled his eyes back, stretched his neck, foamed at the mouth, lay as if dead, and rose up unnaturally. He continued to display extreme, unfocused, and undirected anger, which like Shaw's, functioned simply to satisfy itself. Dudgale predicted the arrival of a preacher named Carrington, who, much to the amazement of those around him, appeared to become a locus for Dugdale's fury. Dugdale 'most furiously raged, threatened to tear him to pieces, struggled most violently to get at him' and 'for an hour poured forth the bitterest Execrations and Blasphemies...Oh Carrington, I hate thee mortally. Oh! I will be revenged on Thee'.[83] Dudgale's fits came often and violently, sometimes manifesting as self harm, and sometimes as strings of inarticulate gibbering, or long stings of expletives, or words in unknown and foreign languages such as Greek and Latin.[84] Rage appeared as a defining feature of Dugdale's possession, and his debates with Carrington fed into the loop continuing throughout the narrative. Apart from raging, Dugdale's fits evolved into athletic dancing, in which he would leap up into the air and dance on his knees and toes, bringing the cycle back to where it began, with a demonic desire to dance.[85]

Richard Dugdale's fits could have been faked - they looked like nights of debauching, dancing, and drinking. They might have been read as St. Vitus' dance, or choreomania (χορεία μανία). In Richard Burton's *Anatomy of Melancholy*, St. Vitus' dance is explained as madness which presents as dancing.[86] However, in their length and voracity, they operated at the far end of human comprehension - which seems a likely place for possession to occur. Dugdale's possession was built on his normal practices (in all likelihood Dugdale had sworn and danced before). However, the language used to describe the extremity of his possession behaviours seems to be reaching for a new way of explaining the common that had become uncommon. He reached near incomprehensible heights: he danced *en pointe* and could suddenly speak Greek and Latin. He reached new depths: his body gruesomely distorted and his speech descended into gibberish. His violence and hatred for Carrington appeared as a kind of too-hot hatred for preachers in general and Carrington in particular. Carrington provided Dugdale an exterior focus for his aggression, but Dugdale's possession was also intensely personal. These two focuses operated iteratively and fed into one another. He raged against Carrington and hurt himself; pain made him angrier and he took that rage out on Carrington. Moreover, his possession was communicative and physical; thoughts translated into action without intermediary treatment. It wasn't just the strength and longevity of Dugdale's rage that marked it as possession: his possession experience was aware of and indifferent to the social structures that condemned and supported it. Cognition is for action. Dugdale did not act without thinking - he thought and performed his possession in tandem and out loud.

Although accompanied by supernatural stillness, stretching, contracting, and contorting, many instances in the above cases look like, and are, performed as normal, albeit extreme, human exclamations and physical displays of anger. These cases share a number of similarities beyond physical and verbal rages: they have haunting moments of silence and stillness, bizarre bodily contortions, and the suggestion of visible and invisible participants guiding, at least in part, the performances. However, the differences between the young maid's warnings, Christian Shaw's arguments, and Richard Dugdale's brawling, suggests that although we cannot know what Dugdale, Shaw, or the maid were so mad about, the physical and conceptual tools used to produce rage in their possessions were in some way individualized and already hardwired from past experience of anger.

Conclusions

Understanding rage possession as ultimately originating within individual experiences of anger also allows us to turn to other spiritual performances, such as moments of great

[79] *Ibid*. 4.
[80] Stemler 2004.
[81] Jollie 1697, 1-2.
[82] Jollie 1697, 3.
[83] *Ibid*. 6.
[84] *Ibid*. 9, 13.
[85] *Ibid*. 32.
[86] Burton 1621, 15.

stillness recorded in both Anglo-Saxon and Early Modern text. Often read as an absenting of the self from the body, these stillnesses might instead have an origin in previous feelings of powerlessness - a withdrawal and retreat into the self, born from social anxiety or insecurity, and made worse by the eyes which watched and the pins which tested the reality of the state of withdrawal. Understanding the physiological, conceptual, and social attributes which contribute to the experience of rage possession offers us a preliminary way to unpack some of what at times seems a surprising onset of vicious ire and violence. The possibility that victims of possession already had experienced enough rage to conjure new experiences of it likewise helps explain the differences which we see in performances of possession: they begin physiologically and conceptually in different personal experiences of anger. Two important and interrelated factors allow rage to become rage possession; the narrative framework and the social support. These narratives are reported, in part, by the communities which gathered around the possessed, watching, empathizing, and perhaps mimicking behaviours. By mirroring aggression back to the possessed, these communities perpetuated a struggle in which authority and submission are negotiated. Rather than drain energy from the possessed, this negotiation potentially fuelled the possession further. Likewise, in gathering and watching, they committed themselves to a position within a narrative in which there is something special and supernatural happening. They produced a story and the possessed feed their faith back into it. These elements could create a space where displays of rage are not only allowed, but, perhaps, (knowingly or unknowingly) encouraged. Rage possession is a consistent, supported, affective snowball: it allows anger to grow by allowing it to pick up aggregate conceptual, physiological, and cultural material.

Rage possession is a constant in the historical evolution of possession in England, from the earliest extant narratives to the copious documents of the Early Modern period. It no doubt also resonates with aspects of historical possession on the continent through these periods, though we have limited the current analysis to two significant time points in a single geographic location. However, with this model, we hope to provide a way to look forward and backwards to trace the similarities in possession experiences by understanding what we innately,[87] cross culturally,[88] and, we propose, trans-temporally, recognize as rage.

Abbreviations

PL Migne, J.P (ed), 1844-64. *Patrologia Latina*, Paris.

Bibliography

Almond, P.C. 2004. *Demonic Possession and Exorcism in Early Modern England*, Cambridge: Cambridge University Press.

Anon., 1619. *The Wonderful Discoverie of the Witchcrafts of Margaret and Phillip Flower*, London: by G. Eld for I. Barnes.

Apps, L. and Gow, A. 2003. *Male Witches in Early Modern Europe*, Manchester: Manchester University Press.

Asch, S. 1985. 'Depression and Demonic Possession: The Analyst as an Exorcist', *Hillside Journal of Psychiatry*, **7.2**, 149-64.

Barrett, L.F. and Lindquist, K.A. 2008. 'The Embodiment of Emotion', in G.R. Semin and E.R. Smith, (eds.), *Embodied Grounding: Social, Cognitive, Affective, and Neuroscientific Approaches*, 237-262, Cambridge: Cambridge University Press.

Barsalou, L.W. 2008. 'Grounding symbolic operations in the brain's modal systems', in G.R. Semin and E.R. Smith, (eds.), *Embodied Grounding: Social, Cognitive, Affective, and Neuroscientific Approaches*, 9-42, Cambridge: Cambridge University Press.

Bede, *In Matthaei Evangelium Expositio* 1.4, *PL* 92, col. 23C.

Boddy, J. 1989. *Wombs and Alien Spirits: Women, Men, and the Zār Cult in Northern Sudan*, Madison: University of Wisconsin Press.

Bonser, W. 1963. *The medical background of Anglo-Saxon England: a study in history, psychology, and folklore*, London: Wellcome Historical Medical Library.

Boroditsky, L. and Prinz, J. 2008. 'What thoughts are made of', in G.R. Semin and E.R. Smith, (eds.), *Embodied Grounding: Social, Cognitive, Affective, and Neuroscientific Approaches*, 98-115, Cambridge: Cambridge University Press.

Boureau, A. (trans. T. L. Fagan) 2006. *Satan the Heretic: The Birth of Demonology in the Medieval West*, Chicago: University of Chicago Press.

Bourguignon, B. 1976. *Possession*, San Francisco: Chandler & Sharp.

Bower, E. 1653. *Doctor Lamb Revived*, London.

Braulio of Saragossa, *Life of Aemilian the Confessor*, *PL* 80.

Burton, R. 1621. *The Anatomy of Melancholy*, Oxford: Printed by Iohn Lichfield and Iames Short, for Henry Cripps.

Caciola, N. 2003. *Discerning Spirits: Divine and Demonic Possession in the Middle Ages*, Ithaca and London: Cornell University Press.

Caciola, N. 2005. 'Breath, Heart, Guts: The Body and Spirits in the Middle Ages', in G. Klaniczay and É. Pócs (eds), *Communicating with the Spirits*, 21-37, Budapest and New York: Central European University Press.

Chajes, J.H. 2001. 'Jewish exorcism: early modern traditions and transformations', in L. Fine, (ed.), *Judaism in Practice, from the Middle Ages through the Early Modern Period*, 386-98, Princeton: Princeton University Press.

Clarke, B. 1975. *Mental disorder in earlier Britain: exploratory studies*, Cardiff: University of Wales Press.

Clark, S. 1997. *Thinking with demons: the idea of witchcraft in Early Modern England*, Oxford: Clarendon Press.

Cohen, E. and Barrett, J.L. 2008. 'Conceptualizing Spirit Possession: Ethnographic and Experimental Evidence', *Ethos*, **36**, 246–267.

Colgrave, B. and Mynors, R.A.B. (eds), 1969. *Bede's Ecclesiastical History of the English People*, Oxford: Clarendon Press.

[87] Ekman 1972.

[88] Elfenbein and Ambady 2002, esp. 222.

Colgrave, B. (ed.), 1956. *Felix's Life of Saint Guthlac*, Cambridge: Cambridge University Press.

Collier, M. 2005. 'Hume and Cognitive Science: The Current Status of the Controversy over Abstract Ideas', *Phenomenology and the Cognitive Sciences*, **4**, 197–207.

Conway, M.D. 1881. *Demonology and Devil-Lore*, 2 vols., New York: H. Holt.

Crislip, A. 2005. 'The Sin of Sloth or the Illness of the Demons? The Demon of Acedia in Early Christian Monasticism', *Harvard Theological Review*, **98.2**, 143-69.

Cullen, Lord F. G. 1698. *Sadducimus Debellatus: Or, a True Narrative of the Sorceries and Witchcrafts Exercis'd by the Devil and his Instruments upon Mrs. Christian Shaw, Daughter of Mr. John Shaw, of Bargarran in the County of Renfrew in the West of Scotland, from Aug. 1696 to Apr. 1697*, London: Printed for H. Newman and A. Bell; at the Grasshopper in the Poultry, and at the Crosse Keys and Bible in Cornhill near Stocks-Market.

Dendle, P. (forthcoming). *Demon Possession in Anglo-Saxon England*. Medieval Institute Publications: Western Michigan University.

Deren, M. 1953. *Divine Horsemen: the Living Gods of Haiti*, New York: Vanguard Press.

Dwyer, G. 2003. *The Divine and the Demonic: Supernatural Affliction and its Treatment in North India*, London and New York: Routledge Curzon.

Ekman, P. 1972. 'Universal and Cultural Differences in Facial Expression of Emotion', in J.K. Cole (ed.) *Nebraska Symposium on Motivation, 1971*, vol. 19, 207-282, Lincoln: University of Nebraska Press.

Elfenbein, H.A. and Ambady, N. 2002. 'On the Universality and Cultural Specificity of Emotion Recognition: A Meta-Analysis', *Psychological Bulletin*, **128**, 203-235.

Fear, A.T. (trans.) 1997. *Lives of the Visigothic Fathers*, Liverpool: Liverpool University Press.

Ferracuti, S., Sacco, R. and Lazzari R. 1996. 'Dissociative Trance Disorder: clinical and Rorschach findings in ten persons reporting demon possession and treated by exorcism', *Journal of Personality Assessment*, **66**, 525-39.

Ferrari, P.F., Gallese, V., Rizzolatti, G. and Fogassi, L. 2003. 'Mirror neurons responding to the observation of ingestive and communicative mouth actions in the monkey ventral premotor cortex', *European Journal of Neuroscience*, **17:8**, 1703-1714.

Freud, S. 1923. 'Eine Teufelsneurose im Siebzehnten Jahrhundert', *Imago*, **9**, 1-34.

Gannon, T.A. 2009. 'Social Cognition in Violent and Sexual Offending: an Overview'. *Psychology, Crime & Law*, **15**, 97-118.

Glenberg, A.M. 2008. 'Toward the integration of bodily states, language, and action' in G.R. Semin and E.R. Smith, (eds.), *Embodied Grounding: Social, Cognitive, Affective, and Neuroscientific Approaches*. 43-70, Cambridge: Cambridge University Press.

Goff, D., Brotman A. and Kindlon, D. *et al.* 1991. 'The delusion of possession in chronically psychotic patients', *Journal of Nervous and Mental Disease*, **179**, 567-71.

Gonser, P. (ed.) 1909. *Das angelsächsische Prosa-Leben des hl. Guthlac*, Heidelberg: Carl Winter's Universitätsbuchhandlung.

Goodcole, H. 1621. *The Wonderfull Discouerie of Elizabeth Sawyer*, London: Printed by A. Mathewes for William Butler, to be Sold at his Shop in Saint Dunstons Church-yard, Fleetstreet.

Goossens, L. 1974. *The Old English Glosses of MS. Brussels, Royal Library, 1650 (Aldhelm's De Laudibus Virginitatis), edited with an introduction, notes, and indexes*, Brussels: Paleis der Academiën.

Greenfield, S. (ed.) 2008. *Spirits with Scalpels: The Cultural Biology of Religious Healing in Brazil*, Walnut Creek, CA: Left Coast Press.

Hale, A. and Pinninti, N. 1994. 'Exorcism-resistant ghost possession treated with Clopenthixol', *British Journal of Psychiatry*, **165**, 386-388.

Hopper, Mrs. 1679. *Strange News from Arpington near Bexly in Kent*, London: Printed for Benjamin Harris.

Henderson, J. 1982. 'Exorcism and possession in psychotherapy and practice', *Canadian Journal of Psychiatry*, **27**, 129-34.

Hurston, Z.N. 1938. *Tell My Horse*, New York: HarperCollins.

Jackson, S.W., 1986. *Melancholia and Depression: From Hippocratic Times to Modern Times*, New Haven and London: Yale University Press.

Jollie, T. 1697. *The Surey Demoniack, or, An Account of Satans Strange and Dreadful Actings, in and about the Body of Richard Dugdale of Surey, near Whalley in Lancashire and How He was Dispossest by Gods Blessing on the Fastings and Prayers of Divers Ministers and People...* , London: Printed for Jonathan Robinson.

Keller, M. 2002. *The Hammer and the Flute: Women, Power, and Spirit Possession*, Baltimore: The Johns Hopkins Press.

Kemp, S. 1989. "Ravished of a Fiend": Demonology and Medieval Madness', in C. Ward, (ed.), *Altered States of Consciousness and Mental Health: A Cross-Cultural Perspective*, 67-78, New York: Sage Publications.

Keysers, C. and Gazzola, V. 2009. 'The observation and execution of actions share Motor and somatosensory voxels in all tested subjects: single-subject analyses of unsmoothed fMRI data', *Cerebral Cortex*, **19**, 1239-55.

Krusch, B. 1885. *Gregorii episcopi Turonensis miracula et opera minora*, Monumenta Germaniae Historica, Scriptores Rerum Merovingicarum, Book 1, part 2, Hanover: Hahn.

Krusch, B. 1888. *Fredegarii et aliorum chronica; Vitae Sanctorum*, Monumenta Germaniae Historica, Scriptores Rerum Merovingicarum, Book 2, Hanover: Hahn.

Kylie, E. (ed. and trans.) 1911. *The English Correspondence of Saint Boniface: Being for the Most Part Letters Exchanged Between the Apostle of the Germans and His English Friends*, London: Chatto & Windus.

Larner, C. 2002. 'Was witch-hunting woman-hunting?' in D. Oldridge, (ed.), *The Witchcraft Reader*, 273-75, London and New York: Routledge.

Lamm, C.C., Baston, D. and Decety, J. 2007. 'The neural substrate of human empathy: effects of perspective-taking and cognitive appraisal', *Journal of Cognitive Neuroscience*, **19**, 42-58.

Leavitt, J. 1993. 'Are trance and possession disorders?' *Transcultural Psychiatric Research Review*, **30**, 51-57.

Lewis, M. 1970. 'A Structural Approach to Witchcraft

and Spirit-Possession', in M. Douglas, (ed.), *Witchcraft: Confessions and Accusations*, 293-309, London: Tavistock Publications.

Lewis, M. 1971. *Ecstatic Religion: An Anthropological Study of Spirit Possession and Shamanism*, Harmondsworth: Penguin.

Lindsay, W. M. (ed.) 1911. *Isidori Hispalensis Episcopi Etymologiarum sive Originum Libri XX*, Oxford: Clarendon Press.

Lindquist, K.A., Barrett, L.F., Bliss-Moreau, E. and Russell, J.A. 2006. 'Language and the perception of emotion', *Emotion*, **6.1**, 125–138.

M.Y. 1669. *The Hartford-shire Wonder, Or, Strange News from Ware being an Exact and True Relation of one Jane Stretton the Danghter [sic] of Thomas Stretton*, London.

McNamara, J.A. and Halborg J.E. 1992. *Sainted Women of the Dark Ages*, Durham and London: Duke University Press.

McNeill, D. 1992. *Hand and Mind: What Gestures Reveal about Thought*, Chicago: University of Chicago Press.

McNeill, D., Duncan, S.D., Cassell, J. and Levy, E.T. (eds.) 2007. *Gesture and the Dynamic Dimension of Language*, Philadelphia: John Benjamins Publishing Company.

Marco, I., Molnar-Szakac, I., Gallese, V., Buccino, G., Mazziotta, J.C. and Rizzolatti, G. 2005. 'Grasping the intentions of others with one's own mirror neuron system', *Public Library of Science*, **3**, 529-535.

Matlock, T. 2004. 'Fictive motion as cognitive simulation', *Memory and Cognition*, **32**, 1389-1400.

Meaney, A.L. 1992. 'The Anglo-Saxon view of the causes of illness', in S. Campbell, B. Hall and D. Klausner, (eds), *Health, disease, and healing in Medieval Culture*, 12-33, New York: St. Martin's Press.

Newman, B. 1998. 'Possessed by the Spirit: Devout Women, Demoniacs, and the Apostolic Life in the Thirteenth Century', *Speculum*, **73**, 733-70.

Niedenthal *et al.* 2009. *Journal of Personality and Social Psychology*, **96**, 1120 –1136.

Obeyesekere, G. 1981. *Medusa's Hair: an Essay on Personal Symbols and Religious Experience*, Chicago: University of Chicago Press.

Obeyesekere, G. 1984. *The Cult of the Goddess Pattini*, Chicago: University of Chicago Press.

Oesterreich, T.K. 1930. *Possession and Exorcism among Primitive Races, in Antiquity, the Middle Ages, and Modern Times*, New York: R.R. Smith.

Oliphant, R. 1966. *The Harley Latin-Old English Glossary*, The Hague: Mouton & Co.

Petitpierre, Fr. R. (ed.) 1972. *Exorcism: The Report of a Commission Convened by the Bishop of Exeter*, 15-16, New York: SPCK.

Rank, O. 1958. *Beyond Psychology*, New York: Dover.

Roberts, A. 1616. *A Treatise of Witchcraft: Wherein Sundry Propositions are Laid Downe*, Kings-Linne in Norffolke.

Sands, K.R. 2004. *Demon Possession in Elizabethan England*, WestPort: Greenwood Publishing Group.

Schulte-Ruther, M., Markowitsch, H.J., Fink, G.R., and Piefke, M. 2007. 'Mirror neuron and theory of mind mechanisms involved in face-to-face interactions: a functional magnetic resonance imaging approach to empathy', *Journal of Cognitive Neuroscience*, **19**, 1354–1372.

Semin, G.R. and Cacioppo, J. T. 2008. 'Grounding Social Cognition', in G.R. Semin and E.R. Smith, (eds), *Embodied Grounding: Social, Cognitive, Affective, and Neuroscientific Approaches*, 119-147, Cambridge: Cambridge University Press.

Sengers G. 2003. *Women and Demons: Cult Healing in Islamic Egypt*, Boston and Leiden: Brill.

Sluhovsky, M. 2002. 'A divine apparition or demonic possession?' in D. Oldridge, (ed.), *The Witchcraft Reader*, 254-266, London and New York: Routledge.

Stemler, G. 2004. 'Physiological Processes During Emotion', in P. Philippot and R. S. Feldmen (eds), *The Regulation of Emotion*, 33-70, New Jersey: Lawrence Erlbaum Associates Publishers.

Stryker, W.G. 1951. 'The Latin-Old English Glossary in MS Cotton Cleopatra A.iii', unpublished Ph.d. Dissertation, Stanford University.

Suggett, R. 2000. 'Witchcraft dynamics in Early Modern Wales', in M. Roberts and S. Clarke, (eds), *Women and Gender in Early Modern Wales*, 75-103, Cardiff: University of Wales Press.

Tangl, M. 1955. *Die Briefe des Heiligen Bonifatus und Lullus.* Monumenta Germaniae Historica, Epistolae Selectae I, Berlin: Weidmann.

Taylor, G. 1978. 'Demoniacal Possession and Psychoanalytic Theory', *British Journal of Medical Psychology*, **51**, 53-60.

Temkin, O. 1945. *The Falling Sickness: A History of Epilepsy from the Greeks to the Beginnings of Modern Neurology*, Baltimore: The Johns Hopkins Press.

Thomas, K. 1971. *Religion and the Decline of Magic*, London: Weidenfeld & Nicolson.

Thompson, E. 2001. 'Empathy and consciousness', *Journal of Consciousness Studies*, **8**, 1-32.

Toohey, P. 2004. *Melancholy, Love, and Time: Boundaries of the Self in Ancient Literature*, Ann Arbor: University of Michigan Press.

de Vogüé, A. (ed.) 1979. *Dialogues*, vol. 2, Paris: Éditions du Cerf.

Ward, C.A. 1989. 'Possession and exorcism: psychopathology and psychotherapy in a magico-religious context', in C.A. Ward, (ed.), *Altered States of consciousness and mental health: a cross-cultural perspective*, 125-144, Newbury Park, California: SAGE Publications.

Zalta, E.N. (ed.) 2009. *The Stanford Encyclopedia of Philosophy*, Stanford University: http://plato.stanford.edu/

Zimmerman, O.J. (trans.). 1959. *Saint Gregory the Great: Dialogues*, New York: Fathers of the Church.

Zwann, R.A. 2004. 'The immersed experiencer: toward an embodied theory of language comprehension', in B.H. Ross, (ed.), *The Psychology of Leaning and Motivation*, 35-58, San Diego: Elsevier Academic Press.

Chapter Three

Outlawry and Moral Perversion in Old Norse Society

Anne Irene Riisøy

Introduction

Of the many problems connected with the *níðingr* (cowardly person) and the *vargr* (skulking, ravenous wolf), here I will explore the connection between these terms and concepts of outlawry and moral perversion in Old Norse Society (*c.* AD800 to *c.* AD1300).

Unlike today's overall term 'outlawry' in English (or *fredløshet* in the Scandinavian countries), different terms were used to describe various facets of outlawry in Old Norse society. In Norway, for instance, *útlagr*, which means to be placed outside the law with a concomitant loss of legal protection, was a general term.[1] Often we have to rely on the context or additional information to decide whether the outlaw had committed an irredeemable crime, lost his real estate, or whether his crime was morally condemned. For instance, paragraph 314 in the *Old Law of the Gulathing* from Western Norway, which concerns men raiding in longships, illustrates a moral aspect. The raiders were decreed outlaws, but whether they were also branded 'nithings' was dependent upon whether peace was renounced before marauding commenced. This distinction is borne out in formulations like *þa ero þeir utlager. oc niðingar,* 'they are outlaws and nithings too'.[2] Thus it was the lack of public declaration of intent, and the stealthy and unmanly way in which the raiding was done, which made it reprehensible.

Sources

Before I proceed further, it is necessary to make a few remarks on the sources I use (predominantly legislation), and how I use them. A provincial law was the law of an independent region of jurisdiction regardless of its political adherence, and in Scandinavia the provincial laws of Norway (from the Gulathing, the Frostathing, the Eidsivathing and the Borgarthing, henceforth abbreviated G, F, E and B) are the oldest which have been preserved. The raiding men described above appear in a law which was probably first written down in the 11th century - whether early or late is still debated - and which may contain some sections that go further back in time.[3] The earliest fragments date from the late 12th century, and a fairly complete redaction dates from the mid-13th century.[4] Whether we use legislation, sagas, or poetry, the methodological problem is essentially the same. Because the majority of manuscripts date from the 13th and 14th centuries, how can they possibly have anything at all to say about society before this time? According to the 19th century *Germanenrechtschule*, these sources in fact said quite a lot, not only about Old Norse society, but they could also be used to fill in blanks in the history of 'the Germans', whether Tacitus's Germans or the Germans of early Frankish law. Because 'the Germans' belonged to the same *Volksgeist*, circumstances of time and place were irrelevant. Following this theory, the medieval Nordic laws were considered the purest variety of ancient Germanic law, because they were unspoilt by contact with the Roman world. *Níðingsverk* was thus considered an ancient Germanic legal term with a definite application to a certain class of outrageous offences, and *vargr* was the 'gemein-germanishcen Namen des Friedlosen'.[5] The notion, closely associated with German National Socialist ideologies of the 1930s and '40s, that the medieval Nordic laws represent age-old law that had disappeared centuries ago from the more southerly Germanic peoples, no longer has currency. On the other hand, the hypercritical point of view presented by Elsa Sjöholm has, for various reasons, also been dismissed. According to Sjöholm, the Nordic laws are built upon a scholarly tradition and foreign ideology - Christianity. Therefore they can at best only tell something about the society contemporary with the time they were written down.[6] Several scholars have strongly opposed her arguments. Sverre Bagge called attention to the fundamentally unsound method adopted by Sjöholm. Because she has compared a fairly limited number of provisions of Nordic law with a narrow and selected range of non-Nordic legal sources, virtually anything can be proven.[7] Besides, the strength of oral traditions in illiterate societies was not taken into consideration; runic and archaeological evidence was not used; and the idea that a law may consist of several chronological strata was rejected.[8]

The arguments in favour of identifying some laws, or sections of law, as older than others, are persuasive. Besides, contemporary runic inscriptions from Scandinavia and comparison with Anglo-Saxon England have shown that it is possible to use these sources to discuss late Viking-Age and Early Medieval society of the north. In terms of the Anglo-Saxon connection, from the 19th century onwards a range of studies have argued for a definite Scandinavian influence on late Anglo-Saxon law as a result of the Viking invasions of the 9th and 10th centuries.

1 Storm and Hertzberg 1895, 676
2 Keyser and Munch 1846, 103; Larson 1935, 198-199
3 Helle 2001, 17-23; Robberstad 1974, 1-26; Rindal 2004, 108-110
4 Eithun et al. 1994, 12-26
5 Heusler 1911
6 Sjöholm 1988, 50, 250-251
7 Bagge 1988, 500-507
8 Brink 2002, 87-110; Sundqvist 2002, 310-311

Níðingr and *níð*

Níðingr and *vargr* can be hard to define and difficult to translate in a few words. There is a semantic connection between *níðingr* and *níð* which is frequently discussed in relation to the Norse genre of *níðvísur* or *níð*-verse. The *níðingr* was someone who had contravened important ethical rules, committed shameful acts, or behaved as a coward, whereas *níð* is an assertion that a person had performed such an action or might think of doing so. Although *níð* expressed a charge of unmanliness and homosexual perversion, the relevant episodes in the sagas are predominantly about phallic aggression and not homoeroticism.[9] The passive partner is described as contemptible and unmanly, and often it seems that he had previously neglected to avenge a wrong or rise to a challenge, whereas the active partner is not stigmatised to the same extent.

In a society where the warrior ideal prevailed, an accusation of lack of masculinity or lack of assertiveness could have dire consequences. Someone harassed by *níð*-verse had to prove that he was fit to remain within society. Either he behaved as a man in the system of Norse ethic, where the right conduct was, of course, to rise to the challenge; or, as several episodes in the sagas attest, the coward was pronounced every man's *níðingr*.[10] A man could retaliate with impunity if someone composed infamous *níð*-verse about him, according to *Grágás* (a collection of the earliest Icelandic laws first written down in 1117/18) and the oldest laws of the Gulathing and the Frostathing.[11] Indeed, he was expected to take revenge. G paragraph 186 states that a person had the right to compensation only three times, unless he had avenged the wrong in the meantime.[12] Although pecuniary compensation was a legal option, it was considered less honourable. As an illustration of these 'ethics of revenge', Per-Edwin Wallén points to episodes in the sagas where people complain that they do not want to carry their murdered relatives in their purse.[13]

Morality refers to an ideal code of conduct, which would be preferred to the alternatives by all 'right-minded' people in a specific culture, and morality also influences law and concepts of crime and punishment. Unassertive, cowardly behaviour was perceived to be a serious deviation from the prevailing norm in Old Norse society, and thus a perversion. Considering all the negative connotations associated with *níð*, it makes sense that a person who had committed a wrong under such circumstances, and by such methods as to give him the character of an unmanly and deceitful wretch, was designated a *níðingr*. It is possible that the Vikings also exported these ideas. Paul Vinogradoff points out that moral disapproval exercised influence on late Anglo-Saxon criminal law in two ways; mainly through the influence of the Church, which considers crime primarily as a sin, but also through the highly-trained invading Scandinavian warrior elites and their concept of *níð* which asserted that some misdeeds were unworthy of a warrior.[14] Judith Jesch supports and elaborates Vinogradoff's view; adding that this concept of honour and loyalty within the group also applied to the armed merchants of late Viking Age Scandinavia.[15]

In legal usage, the *níðingr* and the *vargr* were occasionally interchangeable, thus at least to a certain degree their deplorable personalities converged. In what follows the term *vargr* will be used throughout, because in references to this creature, translation and interpretation tend to go hand in hand. Some prefer the literal translation, 'warg', others favour 'exile', 'outlaw', or the very interpretive 'strangler', 'werewolf' and even 'demon', while, for instance, the more neutral term 'outcast' is chosen in the English translation of *Grágás*.[16]

Vargr

Poetry and law in Old Norse society were in much closer contact than today,[17] and in late Viking age poetry the image of the skulking ravenous *vargr* feeding on corpses also had legal connotations.[18] Snorri Sturluson's Prose Edda, the *Skáldskaparmál* or 'language of poetry', systematises the concepts of poetical words, including *vargr*: 'It is correct to paraphrase blood or carrion in terms of the beast which is called Strangler, by calling them his Meat and Drink; it is not correct to express them in terms of other beasts. The Strangler is also called Wolf'.[19] *Vargr*, which is rendered 'Strangler' in Arthur G. Brodeurs' translation, was clearly an ambiguous term; *úlfr* as well as *vargr* could refer to the animal wolf, but a semantic difference is that *vargr* also designated a monster.

While some scholars consider the association between the image of the wild wolf hunted by all, and the *vargr* and outlaw, as symbolic, others like Mary Gerstein argue that there was more than an allegorical association.[20] I think it is important to underline that whether a physical transformation from man to beast actually took place is not important. What matters is whether Viking-age and early medieval people actually believed it was possible. A host of studies have demonstrated that the demarcation lines between animals and people, and between people and other super-natural creatures, were blurred. Perhaps the most famous manifestation are the shape-shifters, warriors changed into wolves in battle.[21] But *vargr* was applied to a particular subclass of outlaw who had committed odious crimes. Thus the outlaw was originally no popular hero, but one whose deeds polluted the community so much that he was considered a monstrous evildoer - someone who was 'not human'. It is probably significant that the Old Norse word for the animal itself, wolf (*úlfr*), is never chosen in the legal terms designating outlaws, probably because it was not strong enough or precise enough.

---

9 Meulengracht Sørensen 1983, 27; Lilliequist 2001 *passim*
10 Meulengracht Sørensen 1983, 30-32
11 Keyser and Munch 1846, 70, 225
12 Keyser and Munch 1846, 68; Larson 1935, 140
13 Wallén 1962, 245
14 Vinogradoff 1908, 10
15 Jesch 2001, 258-261
16 Dennis et al. 1980, 184-185; Finsen 1852, 206
17 Lehman 1969, 232; Gurevich 1973, 81
18 Jacoby 1974: 116-121
19 'Vargr heitir dyr; þat er at keNa vic bloð e(ða) hrae sva, at kalla verþ hans e(ða) drykk; eigi er rett at kenna sva við fleiri dyr. Vargr heitit ok vlfr ...' Jacoby 1974, 116-118, Brodeur 1916, 208
20 Gerstein 1974, 133-134; Keyser and Munch 1846, 70, 225; Finsen 1852, 183-185
21 Higley 2005, 365

The actions of the *níðingr* and the *vargr* were subsumed under the penal concept *níðingsverk* (or alternatively *níðingsvíg*), which in the Vest-Norse area was applied to a certain class of outrageous offences, mostly killings. The oldest of the Swedish provincial laws is the *Västgötalagen*, which was used in Västergötland, the western province bordering on Norway. In the Swedish provincial laws, *niþingsværk* only appears in the oldest version of this law (VgL I), written around 1220, in the section of *Orbotämal* which means irredemable and permanent outlawry.[22] G preferred the term *níðingsvíg*, 'nithingkilling', which, according to paragraph 178, includes violent housebreaking (*heimsokn*), burning another to death (*brenner mann inni*) and murdering a man (*myrðir mann*), killing one to whom he has given pledges of safety (*vigr trygða mann sinn*), or one to whom he has given protection or sanctuary (*vigr mann i griðum*); or taking revenge for thieves.

The punishment, which includes irredeemable outlawry and loss of all property, underlines the severity of these crimes. VgL I makes it explicitly clear that when a new king made his tour around the kingdom, he had the power to grant outlaws a reprieve, but not outlaws who had committed nithingdeeds.[23] G 178 prescribes outlawry and also adds forfeiture of all property (*firigort hverium penningi fear sins i lande oc lausum eyri*). VgL I formulates a similar pronouncement: *firigiort landi ok lössum öræ*.[24] According to Bo Ruthström, the set expression regarding forfeiture of property probably originated during the reign of king Haakon the Good (c. 920–961), in the Gulathing which was the core area of his kingdom.[25] From the coast it spread all over Norway, due to the need for kingdom-wide execution of sentences for the worst type of crime. It was imperative that a villain who had been outlawed in one legal province was made an outlaw in the whole realm. Stylistic variation in Norse legal language is also influenced by chronology. According to Rune Røsstad, the *Book on Personal Rights* which contains G 178 belongs to the oldest parts of the *Old Law of the Gulathing*, which therefore adds further support for such an early dating of this formula.[26] This set expression would have reached the province of the Vestgöta in the first half of the 11th century at the latest. The linguistic evidence also fits the political and historical context; for instance sagas praise King Haakon as a champion of law and order. Moreover, during his reign there was a period of consolidation, and the Gulathing was also expanded geographically and reorganised.[27]

A cluster of designations pointing towards the *vargr* and the *níðingr* are found in the rules on burials which were enacted in two of the oldest Norwegian Christian laws, probably during the 11th century, following a change of religion. All people who died should be brought to the churchyard for burial, but not suicides and people who had committed heinous acts: evildoers in general (*udaða menn*), traitors (*drottens svica*), murderers (*morðvarga*), truce breakers (*tryggrova*) and thieves are listed in G, while also people who broke temporally or locally limited peace or protection (*griðniðingar*), arsonists (*brænnu vargar)*, and violent housebreakers (*hæimsoknar vargar*) are listed in E.[28]

First in the long list of specific categories denied burial are traitors (*drottens svica*). A *dróttin* was a title for a lord in a broader sense, whether he was a king, leader of a war band, an owner of slaves, and, after the introduction of Christianity, even Christ.[29] According to VgL I it was a nithingsdeed to kill one's *lönær droten* - a term which here refers to the master, in modern Swedish *husbonde*, not the king.[30] A similar sentiment is also expressed in *Grágás, Vígslóði* 102, where the slave who kills his master (*drottne*) or his mistress (*drottningo*) is singled out as one of four outlaws who were particularly reprehensible.[31] To betray one's lord or master was the worst crime imaginable. Based upon contemporary runic inscriptions and skaldic verse, Jesch argues that betrayal was already considered the deed of a *níðingr* in the Viking age when ideally a man showed complete loyalty within his group, a group who formed a partnership in war or in trade.[32] During the 11th century when Scandinavian kingship grew more powerful, concepts of loyalty and treachery moved away from relationships within a more equal group towards a more clearly defined hierarchicy of the king and his subjects. This point of view is also reflected in Norwegian law, for instance F IV 4 explicitly stresses that plotting to deprive the king of land and subjects was the worst form of a nithingdeed, *níðingsverc hit mesta*.[33]

The perpetrator who burned someone to death (*brennir mann inni* according to G 178) was branded a 'fire-*vargr*' (*brennuvargr*) and denied burial in the churchyard. It was not only an excruciatingly painful way to die; it was also derogatory because often the victim had no way of escape and no possibility of fighting his way out. According to Finn Hødnebø it is not made explicitly clear in Norwegian law whether people who set fire to houses did so with murderous intent.[34] G paragraphs 98 and 99 distinguish between fire set by malicious intent or not. However, while a person who caused fire without hostile intent should restore what he had burned down 'to full value', the punishment was indeed severe if the purpose was malicious. If convicted, he was decreed an irredeemable outlaw who had forfeited all his property and he 'shall be called a fire-*vargr*' (*heitir brennuvargr*).[35] This harsh punishment indicates that the perpetrator had done something more then merely burning down an empty dwelling or barn. Swedish legislation, particularly *Östgötalagen*, offers additional support for this interpretation. Someone who set fire to another's house with intent to let him burn 'shall be called a fire-vargr' (*heti kasnar wargher*; *kase* denotes a pile of logs), a compound term which shows similarity to the Norwegian term quoted above.[36] Ragnar Hemmer points out that what made this act heinous was not only the intent to kill people through burning, but an aggravating factor was the stealthy way in which it was done.

[22] Holmbäck and Wessén 1946, 70-74
[23] Holmbäck and Wessén 1946, 109
[24] Schlyter 1827, 23
[25] Ruthström 2003, 103-132
[26] Røsstad 1997, 110-111, 114
[27] Helle 2001, 28-37

[28] G 23; E II 40; Keyser and Munch 1846, 13-14, 405
[29] Storm and Hertzberg 1895, 139-140
[30] Holmbäck and Wessén 1946, 70, 73; Schlyter 1827, 23
[31] Finsen 1852, 178
[32] Jesch 2001, 255-265
[33] Keyser and Munch 1846, 158
[34] Hødnebø, 1956-78, 694-695
[35] Keyser and Munch 1846, 46-47
[36] Schlyter 1830, 43

Normally this secretiveness is not made explicitly clear, but the *Östgötalagen* presumes that the *vargr* was 'stealing' fire into another's house.[37] Although the term 'fire-*vargr*' is not used in *Grágás*, someone who burned other people to death inside their homes was classified as one of the four nastiest outlaws in Iceland.[38]

We encounter yet another murderous *vargr* with a speciality. The compound term *heimsoknar vargar* gives the impression of the stealthy *vargr* who was seeking out someone in order to attack him at home. In early Germanic society the private house was enclosed by a safety zone, where legal protection was supposed to increase. Therefore attack on people at home was particularly reprehensible. Rebecca V. Colman discusses this crime in a wider Western European context, however without including the Norwegian and Swedish sources, and argues that the original meaning of *heimsókn* was a violent attack with intent to kill.[39] There is also every reason to believe that the *heimsoknar vargar* denied burial in E not only caused material damage to houses, but also intended to cause personal injury. This interpretation is supported by G 178 which states that it was a nithingkilling to break into another man's house to attack him and kill him.[40]

Among the various nithingkillings in G 178, murder (*morð*) is also listed, and a *morðvargr* was denied Christian burial. The *morðvargr* in *Grágás* is another of the four irredeemable classes of outlaw (*scogar menn*) who were singled out as particularly reprehensible.[41] A *morð* was a homicide committed in some stealthy way, where the killer concealed the deed and did not take responsibility for it by making public what he had done. The distinction between manslaughter, *víg* (which it was possible to atone for), and murder (which led to irredeemable outlawry) was an old and very important one and it also appears on 11th century runic inscriptions from Scandinavia.[42] The punishment for murder was more severe than for ordinary manslaying, and the murderer could be killed in his turn, without legal consequences.

Exclusion from the living community

In a (pre-) state society the solving of conflicts and enforcement of law depended upon the parties involved keeping to their agreements. Therefore it was paramount that pledges of peace and security, whether temporary or permanent, were kept. In Old Norse society, people who broke such promises or killed someone they had given pledges to were likened to the *níðingr* or the *vargr*, and as we have seen they were also denied burial. *Grið* refers to a limited period of peace and security granted to a law-breaker to enable him to put his affairs in order, or to peace and security that was enforced at certain times and in certain places, such as the assembly, or the way to and from the assembly, or at home.[43] Ideally a limited period of peace and security was followed by permanent peace. *Trygð* means peace or settlement which had been confirmed by oath and it was particularly used in cases of manslaughter and revenge. For instance, someone who broke a peace pledge or who withheld wergeld money was a pledge breaker.[44] If someone accused of breaking a *grið* or a *trygð* was unable to defend himself with a threefold oath, he became an outlaw and therefore was appropriately designated a *griðnidingr* or a *tryggrofi*.[45] According to *Vatnsdæla saga*, a man who failed to come to the site of combat not only became every man's *níðingr*, but he should also bear the name of *griðníðingr*.[46] This clearly implies that a cowardly person was not to be trusted in legal matters either.

The handling and solving of conflicts in Old Norse society involved elaborate spoken procedures, but only a fragment of a *trygða mal* or 'Peace Guarantee Speech' has been preserved from Norway.[47] A formula which has been preserved in *Grágás* is possibly a Norwegian import, and it states that anyone who 'tramples on treaties made or smites at sureties given, he shall be an outcast despised and driven off as far and wide as ever men drive outcasts off...'. Here the outcast who broke the peace guarantee is a *vargr*.[48] Possibly, to some extent this legal formula was also applied in legal practice, as a few episodes in the sagas attest.[49]

The sources portray an unambiguous picture: the *níðingr* and the *vargr* committed morally depraved actions. Therefore they were forever cast out of the society of the living, and they could be killed with impunity by everyone. The answer to the questions who, where, and how, decided whether an action was subsumed under the penal concept of 'nithingdeed' (or nithingkilling) and thus morally condemned. Violent actions against people one owed particular loyalty to, or to whom one had given pledges, and people unable to defend themselves, come into the category of the victims this type of crime. A typical example is the killing of women which VgL I and the sagas attest.[50] Also *valrof*, that is robbery of a man fallen on the battlefield, is evidenced as one of these crimes over a wide area including Anglo-Saxon England, and as early as the 9th century this term occurs twice on the Rök-stone from Östergötland in Sweden, there also clearly referring to war-booty.[51] It was particularly reprehensible to kill people at places where they were supposed to enjoy greater security, at home or at the assembly, or where they were particularly vulnerable, like in the sauna as VgL I mentions.[52] Whether a killing was morally condemned or not was also dependent on how it was done; secretiveness and avoidance of responsibility were strongly disapproved.

A host of technical terms were used to describe violence, mostly killings, in its various facets. However it is interesting

[37] Hemmer 1966, 693-694
[38] Finsen 1852, 178
[39] Colman 1981, 95-110
[40] Keyser and Munch 1846, 66
[41] Finsen 1852, 178
[42] Jesch 1998, 70-71
[43] Storm and Hertzberg 1895, 248-249
[44] F IX 19; G 316-319; Keyser and Munch 1846, 213, 106-109
[45] F V 9; Keyser and Munch 1846, 178
[46] Meulengracht Sørensen 1983, 29-31
[47] G 320; Keyser and Munch 1846, 110
[48] Dennis et al. 1980, 184-185; Finsen 1852, 206
[49] Jacoby 1974, 43, 57; Martina Stein-Wilkeshuis 2002, 167
[50] Holmbäck and Wessén 1946, 70; Meulengracht Sørensen 1983, 76
[51] Jesch 2001, 260; Pons-Sans 2007, 241; Schlyter 1877, 686-687; Keyser and Munch 1846, 66
[52] Holmbäck and Wessén 1946, 70

to note that while the penal concept is coined in *níð*-terms, nithingdeeds or nithingkillings, the perpetrator was often a *vargr* with an area of expertise. The *brennuvarg* or *kasavarg*, *heimsoknarvarg* and *mordvargr* are mentioned above, while in Swedish law a *gorvargher* mutilated and killed another's cattle, ripping living animals so the intestines hung out. This *vargr*-term is also evidenced in a fragment of older secular law from the eastern part of Norway.[53] *Níð* was used as a compound element in words such as *gríðníðingr*, a man who broke a settled peace or agreement. However, *níð* was not used to designate the various kinds of reprehensible killers, possibly because the big flaw in the personality of the *níðingr* is precisely his passivity: he did not rise to a challenge or take revenge. However if he did respond, he behaved in a cowardly or treacherous way. The *níðingr* still had a place within society, although as an unmanly man he was confined to the margins. Although the *vargr* too is portrayed as a skulking and deceitful creature, his violent actions placed him outside the community, both physically and metaphorically. As his name attests, he was a non-human creature.

The *níðingr* and the *vargr* both met with moral disapproval, but an episode from the *Saga of the Ynglings* in *Heimskringla* illustrates a neat distinction between them. One Midwinter, the legendary mid-7th century Swedish king Braut-Onund, his son Ingjald, and many other people assembled at Uppsala for the sacrifices. Ingjald 'set a-going a boys' game' with Ãlf, the son of another Swedish district king, but it turned out that Ingjald was the weaker player. Both boys were six years old, and today we would not be surprised that Ingjald, after having lost, grew so vexed about it 'that he cried bitterly' (*hann grét mjök*). However, when Ingjald's foster father Svipdag heard that Ingjald had fared ill because he was weaker and no match for Ãlf, Svipdag said that was a great shame (*mikil skömm*). Other saga-episodes show that the word *skomm*, 'shame', borders on *níð*, and it designated someone who dared not fight.[54] However, as a king's son, King Ingjald was not without helpers, and his story takes a new twist. The next day the resourceful Svipdag prepared a somewhat unusual barbeque for his foster son. He had cut out the heart of a *vargr* and had it roasted on a spit. Today's slogan; you become what you eat, very much applied in earlier times too. After eating the heart of the *vargr*, Ingjald 'became the most cruel and most ill-natured of men'. Ingjald's nasty and brutish behaviour is evidenced in the ensuing chapters, and apparently arson became his favourite means to expedite foes and rivals. Ingjald's posthumous reputation is aptly summarised in his nickname 'the Wicked' (*hinn illráði*); he had, after all, slain twelve kings - and all by treachery (*sviki alla í griðum*).[55]

In this case the nithing personality had to be reinforced to become a fully fledged *vargr*. The eating of the *vargr*'s heart to bring about this transformation suggests that 'vargishness' was, to some extent, considered to be contagious. This notion sits well with the term *vargdropi*, literally *vargr*-droppling, which designates the child of an irredeemable outlaw whose only inheritance from his *vargr*-father was moral condemnation and non-human status.[56]

Exclusion from the mortuary community

The notion of the non-human perverted outlaw who had to be excluded from society, and placed outside the law, was ingrained in popular custom. After a change of religion to Christianity, a further, ritual exclusion was implemented; the deceased but still irredeemable outlaw also had to be excluded from the society of the Christian dead, the churchyard. The *vargr*-terminology was adapted to ecclesiastical needs when the oldest paragraphs distinguishing between in-groups and out-groups in the churchyard were worked out. It is difficult to say anything about whether dead outlaws had a special outcast status in Old Norse pre-Christian society. However, after a change of religion the impurity of the dead outlaws' bodies did not cease with death: not only were they excluded from the churchyard, they were to be buried far from human habitation.

In Old Norse society the process of Christianization was long. While the oldest Christian cemeteries in, for instance, Norway, date from the 10th century, in the 11th century, heathen burials are still documented.[57] The most suitable place to inhume outlaws banned from burial in consecrated ground was on the shore (*floðar male*) where 'the tide meets the green sod', a stipulation which was retained in mid-13th century Christian laws.[58] Bertil Nilsson points out that this ruling has no parallels in Canon law, and he suggests that this location was chosen to avoid corpses being re-interred in heathen burial mounds.[59] This might have been one rationale - after all, G 23 prohibits burials in 'a mound or heap of stones'.[60] Nilsson puts forward another plausible thought; the inhumations of outlaws mirror their outcast status in life. Thus in death, they did not belong to the earth, neither to the water.[61] But why, exactly, was the shore chosen? It seems that only one episode from the Old Norse sources describes the shore as appropriate for burial. According to *Landnámabók* or *Book of Settlement*, one of the earliest Christians in Iceland expressed her wish to be buried on the shore (*flöðarmálet*) in order to avoid burial in un-consecrated ground. Since the shore was not consecrated either, it was a geographic location which was neutral.

This particular placement of the dead was perhaps not connected with deviant burial in the first place. A recent analysis of Viking Age burials at Kaupang (Skiringssal, Norway's first and oldest city), situated along the coast of South-Eastern Norway, concludes that there were different contemporary concepts relating to death and burials. However, the placement of the burials in the landscape relates to transitional zones, the mountains or to the shore. As boat burials attest, the sea was also somewhat connected to concepts of death. The idea of the 'holy mountain' can be traced in Iceland (*Eyrbyggjasaga*), and is probably a tradition brought

[53] Holmbäck and Wessén 1946, 73; Keyser and Munch 1848, 522-523; Schlyter 1877, 235; Schlyter 1827, 24
[54] Meulengracht Sørensen 1983, 76
[55] Hollander 1999, 36-43

[56] *Grágás*; *ARFA-þÁTTR*; Finsen 1852, 224
[57] Solli 1996 *passim*; Brendalsmo and Stylegar 2001, 5-47; Rolfsen 1981, 128
[58] G 23; E I 50; Keyser and Munch 1846, 13; 392; Larson 1935, 51
[59] Nilsson 1989, 276
[60] Larson 1935, 51-52
[61] Nilsson 1989, 276

over from Norway but later forgotten in the home country.[62] However, after the change of religion when all dead Christians belonged inside the sacred churchyard, the outsiders had to be placed somewhere else, and the shore was after all known for burials. An interesting addition in a manuscript in the *New Christian Law of the Borgarthing* of 1267/68, explains that the shore was chosen for deviant burials so that no one could be desecrated or damaged (*der som ingen er till meins eller skade*), where '*mein*' has meanings like damage, outrage or desecrate.[63] A notion that the sea, washing over the deviant dead, had some cleansing and regenerative effect fits nicely with ideas on purity/impurity found in other cultures too.[64] Furthermore we know that in Early Medieval Norwegian law, water played an important part in the sentencing of sorcerers and witches, who were to be drowned, and sunk to the bottom of the water.[65] Folke Ström lists several examples from the sagas which show that in Norway and Iceland it was common to tie a stone round the neck of the culprit and then push him or her into the water. The practical advantage of the stone was that it facilitated the drowning while at the same time ensuring that the sorcerer would remain at the bottom of the sea or lake.[66] Sexually abused animals were also drowned.[67] Sorcerers as well as sexually abused animals were categories clearly connected to moral perversion or pollution. Some hundreds of years later, possibly due to Biblical inspiration, fire and burning had taken over as the cleansing remedy in such cases. Once upon a time however, water may have played a far bigger part in getting rid of impurities.

Besides, the outlaw may have been buried where he was executed. *Grágás* places the execution of an irredeemable outlaw as well as the burial of his body in one and the same specific location: 'a place beyond bowshot of anyone's homefield wall, where there is neither arable land nor meadow land and from where no water flows to farm'.[68] It seems that also *Grágás* expresses a geographical neutrality or no-mans-land, a place which evades neat classification. Besides, the formulation 'no water flows to farm' might actually fit the description of the shore; water would always flow from the farm to the shore, never the other way round. It is also worthy of note that F XIV 12 points out that the king's bailiff should take a thief to the thing, and from the thing to the shore (*fiöru*) where he should find a man to slay the thief.[69] Although the paragraph does not state that the thief should be buried at the place of execution, the shore, it is perhaps not unreasonable to assume that this is what occasionally happened. Anyway, as outlaws were outcasts in life as well as in death, burial at a liminal place was appropriate.

Unlike for instance in Anglo-Saxon England,[70] separate cemeteries for criminals are not attested in Old Norse society, but during the later Middle Ages this might have changed, perhaps in city-areas with denser population. Archaeological excavations of a cemetery in Skien in Southern Norway, which have recently been published by Gaute Reitan, provide evidence of deviant burials from the period around the Reformation. The cemetery was in use from the late 10th century until approximately 1600. It went out of general use after the Plague in the mid-14th century, but there are indications that it was subsequently used to bury people whose death sentence had been carried out at the town's place of execution, Galgeholmen (i.e Gallows skerry), which was a mere fifty metres away. This place name resembles other places of execution located outside Norwegian towns during the Middle Ages.[71] Three skeletons of people who had been beheaded were excavated, most probably dating back to the Reformation period. Two of the heads were facing downwards; the third had in addition to the beheading also been burnt, and the head had been placed between the legs. The placing of the head between the legs is probably a very ancient and derogatory custom, perhaps to prevent the deceased from returning from the dead.[72] The same chronological layer also yielded five other skulls, nicely arranged in a half-circle. As Reitan explains, it is possible that these skulls, before their burial in the disused cemetery, had been displayed on posts as a warning to others.[73]

Conclusions

In the late Viking age the worst kind of outlaws were declared unmanly or 'not humans' in perpetuity and placed outside the law. With the arrival of Christianity they were not only excluded from the society of the living but also outlawed from the community of the Christian dead, the sacred churchyard. This of course also shows that the *níðingr* and the *vargr* still played an important, although very negative part, in Old Norse society. Gradually, the *níðingr* and the *vargr* faded into oblivion when old moral concepts rooted in a pre-Christian warrior ideology were replaced by Christian morals. For instance, whereas the *níð*-episodes in the sagas with homosexual overtones picture the active part as less reprehensible than the passive part, Christian thinking does not distinguish between the passive and active roles in homosexual relations.[74] Jonas Lillilequist also points out that from the 1300s onwards, there are only vague traces of a living *níð*-tradition in Sweden.[75] The outlaw cast in the image of the *vargr* was also becoming anachronistic, for instance no such episodes occur in the contemporary Icelandic *Sturlunga Sagas*, written by various authors during the 12th and 13th centuries.[76] I have not found outlaws designated in *vargr*-terms or associated with the *vargr* in Norwegian court cases which have been preserved from the late 13th century onwards either.

These changes are part of the legal transformation which took part during the High Middle Ages. In Norway for instance, the *Landslaw* of 1274 establishes a radically new legal framework for settlements of civil cases. With the stroke of a pen the legal possibility of revenge in cases of sexuality and

62 Lia 2001, 116-117
63 NB II 10; Storm 1885, 166; Storm and Hertzberg 1895, 441
64 Douglas 2000, 189-199
65 G 28; Storm 1885, 18
66 Ström 1942, 171-173
67 G 30; Keyser and Munch 1846, 18; Larson 1935, 57
68 Dennis et al. 1980: 30, 236
69 Keyser and Munch 1846, 252-253; Larson 1935, 397-398
70 Reynolds 1997, 33-41; Reynolds 2010

71 Gade 1985, *passim*; Blom 1960, 163-166
72 Riisøy 2009, 92; Knutsen and Riisøy 2007
73 Reitan 2005, 183-184
74 Sørensen 1983, 26
75 Lillilequist 2001, *passim*
76 Ersland 2001, 20

manslaughter was removed. Thus, pecuniary compensation, which had previously been a shameful option, became the only option, and the differences between a man set on revenge and a man opting for less drastic alternatives were no longer so obvious. At the same time a relatively more peaceful society could dispense of the *vargr* and all his variants of non-human brutish behaviour. The medieval state, Kingdom and Church, introduced new concepts primarily based upon Christian ethics, and coined new terms to express crime, punishment and moral perversion.[77]

Bibliography

Bagge, S. 1988: 'Review of Elsa Sjöholm 1988', *Historisk Tidsskrift*, **69**, 500-507.

Blom, G.A. 1960. 'Galge o. galgbacke', *Kulturhistorisk Lexikon för nordisk medeltid*, 163-166, Malmö: Allhems förlag.

Brendalsmo, J.A. and Stylegar, F. 2001. 'Kirkested i 1000 år. Grend, gård og grav i Liknes, Kvinesdal commune i Aust Agder', *NIKU publikasjoner*, **111**, 5-47.

Brink, S. 2002. 'Law and legal customs in Viking Age Scandinavia', in J. Jesch (ed.), *The Scandinavians from the Vendel Period to the Tenth century: an Ethnographic Perspective*, Studies in Historical Archaeoethnology vol. 5, 87-110, Woodbridge: Boydell Press.

Brodeur, A.G. 1916. *The prose Edda: translated from the Icelandic with an introduction by Arthur Gilchrist*, New York: The American-Scandinavian Foundation.

Colman, R.V. 1981. 'Hamsocn: its meaning and significance in Early English Law', *American Journal of Legal History*, **XXV**, 95-110.

Dennis, A., Foote, P. and Perkins, R. (trans.) 1980. *Laws of early Iceland: Grágás, the Codex Regius of Grágás, with material from other manuscripts*. Winnipeg: University of Manitoba Press.

Douglas, M. 2002, repr. *Purity and Danger*, London and New York: Routledge Classics.

Ersland, G.V. 2001. '... *til død og fredløshed* ...' *Fredløysas innhald og funksjon på Island frå 1117 til 1264*. Oslo.

Eithun, B., Rindal, M., Ulset, M. 1994. *Den Eldre Gulatingslova*, Oslo: Riksarkivet.

Finsen, V. 1852. *Grágás, Islændernes Lovbog i Fristatens Tid*, Kjøbenhavn: Berling.

Gade, K.E. 1985. 'Hanging in Northern Law and Literature', *Maal og Minne* **3-4**: 159-183.

Gerstein, M., 1974. 'Germanic Warg: the Outlaw as Werwolf, in G. J. Larson (ed), *Myth in Indo-European Antiquity*, Berkley: University of California.

Gurevich, A.Y. 1973. 'Edda and Law. Commentary upon Hyndlolióð', *Arkiv för Nordisk Filologi*, **88**, 72-84.

Helle, K. 2001. *Gulatinget og Gulatingslova*, Leikanger:Skald.

Hemmer, R. 1966. 'Mordbrand', *Kulturhistorisk Lexikon för nordisk medeltid*, 693-694, Malmö.

Heusler, A. 1911. *Das Strafrecht der Isländersagas*, Leipzig: Duncker & Humblot.

Higley, S.L. 2005. 'Finding the man under the skin: identity, montrosity, expulsion, and the werewolf ', in T. Shippey, (ed), *The Shadow-walkers: Jacob Grimm's Mythology of the Monstrous*, 335-378, Tempe: Arizona: Medieval and Renaissance Texts and Studies.

Hødnebø, F. 1966. 'Mordbrand', *Kulturhistorisk Lexikon för nordisk medeltid*, 694-695, Malmö.

Hollander, L.M. 1999. *Heimskringla: History of the Kings of Norway*, Austin: University of Texas Press.

Holmbäck, Å. and Wessén, E. 1946. *Svenska Landskapslagar. Femte Serien: Äldre Västgötalagen, Yngre Västgötalagen, Smålandslagens Kyrkobalk och Bjärköarätten*, Stockholm: Gebers.

Jacoby, M. 1974. *Wargus, vargr 'Verbrecher' 'Wolf' eine sprach- und rechtsgeschichtliche Untersuchung*, Uppsala: Almqvist and Wiksell.

Jesch, J. 1998. 'Murder and Treachery in the Viking Age', in T. S. Haskett (ed), *Crime and Punishment in the Middle Ages*, 63-85, Victoria, British Columbia: University of Columbia.

Jesch, J. 2001. *Ships and Men in the Late Viking Age: the Vocabulary of Runic Inscriptions and Skaldic Verse*, Woodbridge: The Boydell Press.

Keyser, R. and Munch, P.A. 1846. *Norges gamle Love indtil 1387, I*, Christiania.

Keyser, R. and Munch, P.A. 1848. *Norges gamle Love indtil 1387, II*, Christiania.

Knutsen, G. and Riisøy, A.I. 2007. 'Trolls and Witches', *Arv: Nordic Yearbook of Folklore*, **63**, 42-48.

Larson, L.M. 1935. *The Earliest Norwegian Laws, Being the Gulathing Law and the Frostathing Law*, New York: Columbia University Press.

Lehmann, W.P. 1969. 'On Reflections of Germanic Legal Terminology and Situations in the Edda', in E. C. Polomé (ed), *Old Norse Literature and Mythology, a Symposium*, Austin and London: University of Texas Press.

Lia, Ø. 2001. *'Det rituelle rom. En fortolkende analyse av vikingtidens graver og landskap på Kaupang*, Unpublished Master's thesis, University of Oslo.

Lilliequist, J. 2001. 'Talet om den hotade maskuliniteten i ett historisk perspektiv. Från niding till sprätt', Paper från det 24:e Nordiska Historikermötet i Aarhus 2001, http://aarhus2001.hum.au.dk/rundborde/rundbord5paper2.html

Nilsson, B. 1989. *De sepulturis: Gravrätten i Corpus Iuris Canonici och i medeltida nordisk lagstiftning*, Stockholm: Almqvist & Wiksell.

Pons-Sanz, S.M. 2007. *Norse-Derived Vocabulary in Late Old English Texts: Wulfstan's works, a Case Study*, Odense: University Press of Southern Denmark.

Reitan, G. 2005. 'Fra kokegroper til halshugginger på Faret', *Varia, Kulturhistorisk Museum Fornminneseksjonen*, **58**, 183-184.

Reynolds, A. 1997. 'The Definition and Ideology of Anglo-Saxon Execution Sites and Cemeteries', in G. De Boe and F. Verhaeghe (eds), *Death and Burial in Medieval Europe – Papers of the Medieval Europe Brugge 1997 Conference*, 33-41. Zellik: Instituut voor het Archaeologisch Patrimonium.

Reynolds, A. (2010). *Anglo-Saxon Deviant Burial Customs*, Oxford: Oxford University Press

Riisøy, A. 2009. *Sexuality, Law and Legal Practice and the*

[77] Riisøy 2009, *passim*

Reformation in Norway. Leiden: Brill.

Rindal, M. 2004. 'Dei eldste norske kristenrettane' in J. V. Sigurðsson, M. Myking and M. Rindal (eds), *Religionsskiftet i Norden. Brytinger mellom nordisk og europeisk kultur 800-1200 e.Kr*, Oslo: Senter for studier i vikingtid og nordisk middelalder.

Robberstad, K. 1974. 'Mostratinget 1024 og Sankt Olavs kristenrett: Etter eit fyredrag på Moster 28. juli 1974', *Stensilserie: Institutt for privatrett*, 1-26, Oslo.

Rolfsen, P. 1981. 'Den siste hedning på Agder', *Viking*, **44**, 112-128.

Røsstad, R. 1997. *A tveim tungum: om stil og stilvariasjon i norrønt lovmål*, Oslo: Noregs forskingsråd.

Ruthström, B. 2003. *Land och Fæ. Strukutrellt-rättsfilologiska studier i fornnordiskt lagspråk över beteckningar för egendom i allmänhet med underkategorier*, Lund.

Schlyter, C.J. and Collín, H.S. 1827. *Corpus iuris Sueo-Gotorum antiqui: Samling af Sweriges gamla Lagar, Westgötalagen, I.* Stockholm: Z. Haeggström.

Schlyter, C.J. and Collín, H.S. 1830. *Corpus iuris Sueo-Gotorum antiqui: Samling af Sweriges gamla Lagar, Östgötalagen, II.* Stockholm: Z. Haeggström.

Schlyter, C.J. and Collín, H.S. 1877. *Corpus iuris Sueo-Gotorum antiqui: Samling af Sweriges gamla Lagar, Ordbok XIII.* Stockholm: Z. Haeggström.

Sjöholm, E. 1988. *Sveriges medeltidslagar: europeisk rättstradition i politisk omvandling*. Lund.

Solli, B. 1996. 'Narratives of Encountering Religions: On the Christianization of the Norse around AD 900-1000', *Norwegian Archaeological Review*, **29**, 89-114.

Stein-Wilkeshuis, M. 2002. 'Scandinavians Swearing Oaths in Tenth-century Russia: Pagans and Christians', *Journal of Medieval History*, **28**, 155-168.

Storm, G. 1885. *Norges gamle Love indtil 1387, IV*. Christiania.

Storm, G. and Hertzberg, E. 1895. *Norges gamle Love indtil* 1387, V. Christiania.

Ström, F. 1942. *On the Sacral Origin of the Germanic Death Penalties*, Lund: H. Ohlssons boktryckeri.

Sundqvist, O. 2002. *Freyr's Offspring: Rulers and Religion in Ancient Svea Society*, Uppsala: Uppsala University Press.

Sørensen, P.M. 1983. *The Unmanly Man: Concepts of Sexual Defamation in Early Northern Society*, Odense: Odense University Press.

Vinogradoff, P. 1908. *English Society in the Eleventh Century, Essays in English Medieval History*, Oxford: Clarendon Press.

Wallén, P. 1962. Hämnd, *Kulturhistorisk Lexikon för nordisk medeltid*, 239-246. Malmö.

Chapter Four

Hermaphroditism in the western Middle Ages: Physicians, Lawyers and the Intersexed Person

Irina Metzler

Introduction

Hermaphroditism is not a disease or illness in the modern sense, but it is a condition that has been pathologised by the medical profession and legislated about by the jurists, and has prompted the framing of philosophical questions about personhood and gendered identity. For all its modern connotations, such a statement is equally valid for the medieval period: after all, medieval physicians and surgeons had their attention drawn to the phenomenon of hermaphroditism to the extent of writing about it in their didactic material, while both civil and canon lawyers felt impelled to mention hermaphrodites in their codifications; nor were medieval intellectuals any less prone than their modern counterparts to philosophizing about the meaning of life, in this case about the meaning of people who, although definitely one-hundred-percent human, were nevertheless different enough to arouse some awkward questions about universally-accepted, God-given binaries such as male and female.

In this context, one may compare the condition of being a hermaphrodite to the condition of being (physically) disabled. Both the hermaphrodite and the disabled person are persons in the widest sense, but do not neatly fit into the binary categories so beloved of western, medieval as well as modern, society. The situation in medieval Islamic societies was different only in so far as the boundary between male and female was drawn even more firmly than in medieval and early modern European societies, so that a person who fitted neither of the available gender categories 'presented a serious dilemma'.[1] To overcome that dilemma, medieval Islamic jurists proposed assigning a gender to such a person at the earliest possible point, for instance shortly after birth in the case of an infant born with ambiguous genitalia.[2] In this respect, they were acting in a thoroughly 'modern' fashion, since today, too, in many western countries, notably the United States, there are endeavours, especially by the medical profession, to assign one or the other binary category from birth. Whereas modern societies primarily rely on medical authorities, medieval Islamic societies relied on jurists, who aimed to ensure socialisation of the ungendered hermaphroditic body. 'What was at stake for medieval Muslims in gendering an ungendered body was, by implication, gendering the most important body: the social body'.[3] How medieval Christian societies reacted to and interacted with hermaphrodite, ungendered bodies will be explored below.

[1] Sanders 1991, 75: I am indebted to Prof. Monica Green for drawing my attention to this article.

[2] *Ibid*, 77.

[3] *Ibid*, 89.

Disabled people are neither truly ill nor are they conventionally healthy (at least according to the medical model of disability, that is), and hermaphrodites are neither female nor male. Both can therefore be regarded as liminal persons:[4] the disabled person occupies a liminal space between health and illness, while the hermaphrodite is situated in a liminal sexual territory. One of the topics this essay will explore is therefore the comparison of, and similarities between, disability and hermaphroditism. Another topic is formed by looking at the differing medieval and modern notions of gender and sex. Hermaphrodites are deemed anatomically abnormal by modern medical discourse. Medieval medical (and philosophical) discourse tried to find ways of accommodating such abnormality, but nevertheless fell far short of the kind of acceptance that the modern term 'intersex' implies. Medieval reactions to hermaphroditism were strongly influenced by fears of social deviance, so much so that such fears actually informed the attempts at categorisation and explanation of the phenomenon of hermaphroditism. Rather than an aberrant physiology, what worried medieval commentators more was the possibility of aberrant sexual, in this case homosexual, behaviour. Medieval discussions of hermaphroditism did not invariably distinguish between the behaviourally deviant (effeminate men/ virago women) and the biologically deviant (differently developed sexual organs), as the modern viewpoint likes to do; instead the medieval boundaries were fuzzy and blurred.

The topic of hermaphrodites has been well-researched for antiquity, for example by Luc Brisson,[5] who brings together and translates most texts on the subject besides the familiar sources of Ovid's *Metamorphoses* (4.285-388) and Plato's *Symposion*. At the other end of the timeline, hermaphrodites in the Renaissance and early modern period have been discussed in the work of Lorraine Daston and Katherine Park, for example, in their early essay 'Hermaphrodites in Renaissance France'.[6] But the medieval period, as so often, falls between the stools of scholarly attention. Besides an article by Miri Rubin on hermaphrodites published in 1996, there has been no more recent single thematic publication. This present article will try to address the gaps, by looking at attitudes and reactions to hermaphrodites in the middle ages, uncovering some of the origins of these reactions in philosophical and medical/ biological ideas of the period, and exploring the extent to which a discourse of modern disability studies is appropriate for discussing medieval hermaphroditism.

[4] Metzler 2006, 31-2.

[5] Brisson 2002.

[6] Daston and Park 1985.

Mediaeval legal interpretations of hermaphroditism

My first encounter with medieval hermaphrodites was not in literary, medical or theological works, but in a legal text. Closer investigation of the context brought to light the notion of personal choice for the hermaphrodite inherent in such texts. This stood in such stark contrast with the modern medical approach of surgical intervention at the earliest opportunity, that it sparked the academic interest which lead to this current piece of research. In the 13th century, the jurist Fleta, associated with Bracton (Henry of Bratton = Henricus de Brattona or Bractona), and commentator on secular law, had the following to say about hermaphrodites:

> Among freemen there may not be reckoned those who are born of unlawful intercourse, such as adultery and the like (by-blow, spurious, bastard) and others begotten of unlawful intercourse, nor those who are procreated pervertedly, against the way of human kind, as for example, if a woman bring forth a monster or a prodigy. Nevertheless, the offspring in whom nature has in some small measure, though not extravagantly, added members or diminished them - as if he should have six fingers or only four - he should certainly be included among freemen. Men may also be classified according to whether they are male or female or hermaphrodite. An hermaphrodite, to be sure, is classed with male or female, according to the predominance of the sexual organs.[7]

In Roman law, in Justinian's *Digest* of the 6th century, the gender status of the hermaphrodite person was already determined by the prevalence of one type of sexual organ:

> *Ulpian*: Question: Whom do we consider an hermaphrodite? I believe that it is to be judged according to the sex which prevails in the person. (*De statu hominum. Ulpianus. Quaeritur: hermaphroditum cui comparamus? et magis puto ejus sexus aestimandum, qui in eo praevalet*).[8]

Here we can immediately identify the main themes of medieval hermaphroditism: the categorisation of licit and illicit, monster or natural, supported by definitions of what constitutes these categories, and the ascription of one single sex to the hermaphrodite. In the legal text compiled during the 1220s and 30s commonly known as *Bracton* itself, the *Fleta* text is abbreviated to read:

> Another classification of men.
>
> Mankind may also be classified in another way: male, female, or hermaphrodite. Women differ from men in many respects, for their position [better: condition] is inferior to that of men.
>
> Of the hermaphrodite.
>
> A hermaphrodite is classed with male or female according to the predominance of the sexual organs.
>
> (*Alia divisio hominum.*
>
> *Est autem alia divisio hominum quod alii sunt masculi, alii feminae, alii hermaphroditi. Et differunt feminae a masculis in multis, quia earum deterior est condicio quam masculorum.*
>
> *De hermaphrodito*
>
> *Hermaphroditus comparatur masculo tantum vel feminae tantum secundum praevalescentiam sexus incalescentis*).[9]

Therefore, legally, hermaphrodites were assigned to one gender and one gender alone. Although not explicitly stated in these texts, according to other legal codes, as will be seen below, it was the hermaphrodite subject him/herself who did the classification: they were permitted some flexibility or choice as to which gender they would belong to, but they needed to adhere to their decision once it had been taken.

Foucault had already argued that the status of hermaphrodites, as determined by medicine and the law, had for a long time been of a dual nature: for centuries people had simply allowed the hermaphrodite to possess two sexes simultaneously, and only with the 18th century had the rejection of multiple sex led to the assertion that a hermaphrodite must belong to just one.[10] For the middle ages, Foucault briefly outlined civil and canon law. According to Foucault's summary, medieval hermaphrodites were those people with ambiguous sex, where the sexual organs of both male and female were present in variable ratios. In such a case the father or godfather - that is, the person 'naming' the child - had the duty to fix the sex of the infant at the time of baptism. If the circumstances allowed, it was advised by the jurists to opt for that sex which was predominant, which had the 'greater strength', or the 'greater heat'. Later however, on the verge of attaining the age of majority, and when the age of permissible marriage approached, the hermaphrodite was free to choose for him- or her- self whether s/he still wanted to belong to the sex ascribed at baptism, or to prefer the other one. The only subsequent judicial restriction was that henceforth the hermaphrodite must stick to this final chosen sex, and might never switch again. If a hermaphrodite renounced this final chosen sex, they ran the risk of being accused of sodomy. Foucault emphasized that such subsequent changes of mind, and not the primary anatomical mixing of the sexes, had carried with them the majority of judicial condemnations and capital punishments of hermaphrodites in France during the medieval and Renaissance periods.[11]

An example of judicial reaction can be found in the following case: in the Alsace, at Breisach in 1281, a female hermaphrodite (*hermaphrodita*) was punished by blinding after s/he had 'violently tried to have sex with a woman' (*Hermaphrodita exocculatur in Briasco, pro eo quod violenter voluit cognoscere mulierem*).[12] This person, described as a hermaphrodite in the female role, was presumably regarded as lapsed in their decision as to which sex and gender role they were to occupy, because they behaved in a distinctly male fashion. What

[7] Fleta in Richardson and Sayles 1955, 60; Damme 1978, 7.

[8] Justinian in Krüger 1971, 35, book 1, tit. 5, 5, and Rubin 1994, 104 note 24.

[9] Bracton in Thorne 1997, 31-2.

[10] Foucault 1998, 7-8.

[11] *Ibid*, 8.

[12] Rubin 1994, 104 note 22, citing the Scriptores 1828, 208, published Hannover: Hahn.

confused medieval contemporaries would have been not so much the hermaphrodite *per se*, but the behavioural deviance, in this case a person defined as female behaving like a male. The reverse, where a person defined as male acts inappropriately as a female, also caused concern. The case of a person who was ostensibly a man but behaved in a distinctly female fashion has recently come to the attention of modern scholars. In 1354, one Rolandino/Rolandina Ronchaia was arrested in Venice. He was married to a woman, but claimed he:

> never knew her or any other woman carnally, because he never had any carnal appetite, and his virile member could never become erect ... and since he was feminine in face, voice, and behaviour, even though he did not have a female orifice and had the member and testicles of a man, many people thought him to be a woman because of his external features.[13]

He may well have been intersex in modern terms, because he also had 'breasts like a woman'. He was noticed by the law because he started dressing like a woman and became a prostitute, having sex with men, during which he 'hid his member' which never became erect as he himself attested. It seems that what worried his 14th-century contemporaries more than his dubious physiology was his taking on the wrong gender role - again, like in the earlier 13th-century case, a behavioural and not a biological issue.

The matter of choice for the hermaphrodite was, in fact, not as totally free as Foucault leads one to believe. Instead, the physically mature hermaphrodite could choose which sex *predominated* for him or her, since it was one's 'nature' that attracted one to the 'opposite sex'.[14] The hermaphrodite was therefore allowed to choose only within the limitations of what contemporaries thought of as their true being or nature. One important aspect of this albeit limited choice, is, however, that the individual could be depended upon to make the choice themselves during the medieval period, without 'further consultation of authorities',[15] be they medical, religious or legal. It was only with the 16th century that legal practice called for 'increasing reliance on outside testimony to determine the hermaphrodite's predominant sex' and the individual hermaphrodite's self-assessment was no longer sufficient.[16]

Popular sterotypes

Because of the gender fluidity and sexual ambiguity that hermaphroditism potentially presented, it could be perceived as dangerous. Hence lawyers, as one group of people reinforcing social and cultural norms, insisted that hermaphrodites should show only one face in front of the law, male or female.[17] Such alleged two-facedness went beyond legal matters and into the realm of popular stereotyping. In a late-medieval medical text, the *Placides et Timéo ou Li secrés as philospohes*, which survives in eight manuscripts dating to between 1304 and the end of the 15th century, a figure called 'Hermaphrodite' surfaces as a devious character, a man who dresses like a woman so as to pass as a female with the aim of infiltrating women's company so that he can learn their secrets.[18] Notions about the danger of sexual or social ambiguity, of course, also found their expression in more literate texts. The perceived fear of anyone who was not really what they appeared to be is exemplified in Eustache Deschamps's (c. 1346-c. 1406) ballad *Contre les hermaphrodites*:

> A soft chin, son Hermaphrodite
> Effeminate, a defect of nature,
> Faint in heart, devoid of all virtues,
> But full of vice, which tends towards nothing but filth,
> A masculine name, a female body
> who are wont to impose false names on others
> I never read the books of such as them
> who are not perfect in nature,
> Corrupt in body, in thought, the pigs,
> untrustworthy, disloyal, evil.
> ... A woman out of a man, who should be bearded,
> man without hair, this is an insult to everyone.
> To meet them is nothing but misfortune,
> And their gaze can be pleasing to no one.
> they make (sexual) use of both kinds,
> I have known them in my time to be
> Untrustworthy, disloyal, evil.[19]

One can compare this with the rhetorical condemnation of corrupt grammar and linguistic style by Alan de Lille in *De planctu naturae* (composed before 1203). This is a homophobic treatise which complains that Venus has turned aside from her role of ensuring reproduction and instead encourages humankind to enter into unnatural forms of intercourse:

> [W]hen Venus wars with Venus and changes 'hes' into 'shes' [sic]...
>
> A man turned woman blackens the fair name of his sex. The witchcraft of Venus turns him into a hermaphrodite. He is subject and predicate: one and the same term is given a double application.
>
> *([0431A] Cum Venus in Venerem pugnans, illos facit illas ...*
> *[0431B] Femina vir factus, sexus denigrat honorem,*
> *Ars magicae Veneris hermaphroditat eum.*
> *Praedicat et subjicit, fit duplex terminus idem,*
> *Grammaticae leges ampliat ille nimis.*)[20]

For Alan de Lille, to 'confuse genders was a corruption of

[13] Karras 2005, 143, citing the manuscript at Archivio di Stato, Venice, Signori di Notte al Criminal, R.6, f.64.
[14] Daston and Park 1996, 124.
[15] *Ibid.*
[16] *Ibid.*
[17] Hadley 2001, 185.

[18] Green 2000, VI 161 and note 57.
[19] Rubin 1994, 105 note 29, citing Saint-Hilaire 1889, 49-50; Rubin also mentions the *Kalendrier des bergiers* for similar sentiments (Rubin 1994, 106 note 30).
[20] Alan of Lille in McCarthy 2004, 177-8. The Latin version is available at http://www.thelatinlibrary.com/alanus/alanus1.html (accessed 14 February 2010).

the nature of language'.[21] Grammar here stands in the same relationship to physiological nature as does the microcosm of the human body in relation to the macrocosm of created nature.

Intellectual discourse is one thing, but popular reaction might be something quite different. As Dawn Hadley suggests, medieval contemporaries 'were not always as accommodating as ecclesiastical, legal or scientific authors, and hermaphrodites were likely to be condemned and shunned'.[22] In simplified terms, scientific and medical texts sometimes described hermaphrodites as occupying an in-between or liminal position, but 'legal and social decisions (ones often arising out of sodomy trials) were made to allocate hermaphrodites to one gender or the other, with the expectation that they would adopt the behaviour of the gender to which they were assigned'.[23] Legal frameworks therefore echoed social expectations of correct behaviour.

Nevertheless, part of Foucault's interpretation is corroborated by the medieval textual evidence. As Joan Cadden has pointed out, hermaphrodite was a wide category that could be construed to mean, in a narrow sense, a person who possesses genital organs proper to both sexes, or, more broadly, a manly woman or a womanly man. Many medical writers of the middle ages thought of hermaphrodites 'as being at one point on a scale between male and female',[24] and manly women or womanly men occupied other points further along the same scale.[25] As Cadden put it: 'The existence of hermaphrodites, accounted for by the same sorts of natural causes [as virile women or effeminate men], likewise suggested that sex definitions and their attendant gender implications *might admit of degrees* [my emphasis], thus disclosing an apparent tension ... between scientific principles, on the one hand, and Christian concerns and lay perspectives, on the other'.[26] If one revisits Foucault's theory of the dual nature permissable to pre-modern hermaphrodites, and their right to possess two sexes simultaneously, then in my interpretation of these degrees of gender Foucault's supposition gains a greater element of plausibility.

Hermaphrodites, sexuality and monstrosity

Hermaphrodites however can deceive: they can use their possession of both male and female sexual characteristics to act female one moment, male the next.[27] 'Both the sexual ambiguity of persons of this sort,' and the possibility they presented of ambiguous sexual pairing, 'led to an association of hermaphroditism with homosexual desires and acts in medieval culture'.[28] Much of the material amassed by John Boswell would imply that in the medieval period homosexuality is conflated with hermaphrodites and eunuchs.[29] Cadden is careful to insist on the fact that the connection between hermaphroditism and homosexuality is still a conjectural one, as it has not yet been solidly documented in medical or scientific sources. Interestingly, elsewhere Cadden cites an early 14th-century commentary by Peter of Abano on the *Problemata* of Aristotle as an example of such a text where natural homosexuality (that is, men for whom anatomical or biological, that is physiological, explanations, can be made for their desire of anal stimulation) is perhaps monstrous, but in the same sense as a hermaphrodite has a 'monstrous nature', which nevertheless conveys 'the sense of an occurrence of and in nature'.[30] From the late 14th century onwards, 'hermaphrodite' becomes a more frequently used term for homosexual, mainly employed by intellectuals in a pejorative sense. For example in his *Bellifortis*, Conrad Kyeser of Eichstätt lambasts king Sigismund of Hungary, calling him the 'king and hermaphrodite of Hungary', because he behaved in an effeminate and cowardly fashion by fleeing the scene after he had lost the battle of Nicopolis (1396).[31] Late medieval normative concepts, or mindsets, could easily interpret hermaphroditism as a form of homosexuality,[32] and it could also be viewed as 'a symbol of Jewish perfidy, say in the context of medieval bestiaries describing the sexual ambiguity of hyenas'.[33] Confusion between homosexual and hermaphroditic phenomena is still apparent in the secondary literature on medieval sources. Chaucer's figure of the Pardoner, for example, is variously interpreted as a eunuch, a hermaphrodite, or a homosexual.[34] Philosophically, in modern interpretation of medieval text and imagery,

> 'the hermaphrodite sculpted in cathedral decorations, painted in liturgical illuminations, and reported in the [ninth-century] *Book of Monsters* and other texts is a contradiction of more than gender distinctions within biology, and it denies more than logical principles: the hermaphrodite is the third term reaching out to join contraries and bringing nonbeing side by side with being, showing through its deforming combination the meaning of that which is and is-not'.[35]

The hermaphrodite cancels sexual pairs, and is thereby disrupting orderly elements. The unequivocalities of the sexual body disappear in the monster, according to modern scholarly criticism of medieval texts, and these presumed clear-cut distinctions instead oscillate between male and female. For example, Ulrich von Utzenbach composed an *Alexanderroman* sometime between 1270 and 1286. According to one interpretation current among modern literary critics he used Alexander's adventures in the East to explore constructions of gender and sexuality in his encounters with monsters.

> In the monster the demonstrative signs of the sexed body are blurred: they oscillate between male and female, as among the bearded women, they turn into monstrous

[21] Rubin 1994, 106.
[22] Hadley 2001, 185.
[23] Garton 2004, 73.
[24] Hadley 2001, 185.
[25] Cf Cadden 1993, 220-7.
[26] *Ibid*, 203.
[27] As in a text *Hermaphroditus* by Antonius Beccadelli, also known as Panormita (1394-1471), published by Frider. Carol. Forbergius-Coburgi Sumtibus Meuseliorum (1824), Bk. II, cap. 37.
[28] Cadden 1996, 63.
[29] Boswell 1980.
[30] Cadden 1997, 47.
[31] cf. Hergemöller 1992, 31.
[32] Rubin 1994, 101-7.
[33] Bildhauer and Mills 2003, 12; on hyenas cf. Hassig 1995, 145-55.
[34] Kuefler 1996, 290.
[35] Williams 1996, 59.

constructs such as the pig-like women, or they become mixed with bestial members as in the Cynocephali [= dog-headed people] so that they do not permit any sex.

> *(Im Monstrum verwischen sich die Eindeutigkeiten des geschlechtlichen Körpers (sex): sie oszillieren zwischen Mann und Frau wie bei den bärtigen Frauen, werden zu monströsen Gegenbildern, wie bei den schweineartigen Frauen, oder vermischen sich, wie bei den* konocefalî, *so mit ihren tierischen Anteilen, daß sie kein Geschlecht zulassen).*[36]

For all the references to hermaphrodites being allowed to switch sex or choose gender, one must remember that these were exceptions ratifying the rule, the rule being two sexes which were regarded as the natural state. Any deviation from this rule was potentially a monstrosity. Augustine in the *City of God* included hermaphrodites in his list of monstrous races, where he says of the Androgyni that they: 'have the characteristics of both sexes, the right breast being male and the left female, and in their intercourse they alternate between begetting and conceiving'.[37] Slightly later in the same chapter Augustine expands some more on this topic:

> As for *Androgynes*, also called Hermaphrodites, they are certainly very rare, and yet it is difficult to find periods when there are no examples of human beings possessing the characteristics of both sexes, in such a way that it is a matter of doubt how they should be classified. However, the prevalent usage has called them masculine, assigning them to the superior sex; for no one has ever used the feminine names, *androgynaecae* or *hermaphroditae*.[38]

Augustine saw the purpose of such anomalies as defining the norm, since by their very rarity they demonstrated what constituted the persistent norm or nature.[39]

The hermaphrodite, too, like other so-called monsters, attains meaning mainly by context. 'The principal difference between prodigies and marvellous species lay in their signification rather than their form'.[40] Thus, in medieval thought, the monstrous races, of whom the African Androgynes were one example, have no intrinsic meaning (beyond an allegorical one), they simply exist, along with all sorts of other natural phenomena, whereas the individual monster, or in this case, the hermaphroditic person, could be treated as a signifier of God's will.

At the same time, however, the androgynous or bisexual could be seen as something positive. Plato, in the *Symposium*, while telling the story of giants who were originally androgynous, but made war on the gods and were defeated and punished by being divided into male and female, so that these weakened creatures then become human men and women,[41] had explained that all present human sexual desire stems from the primordial wish to attain oneness and to re-unite with the former other half that humans once had. Humanity's original state was, according to this text also circulated in the middle ages,[42] one of hermaphroditic dual sex. There are also Judaeo-Christian religious beliefs in the unity of God as meaning sexual unity of God: Adam was therefore created bisexually. References to this can be found in texts by Philo and by Tertullian.[43]

Philo had looked at the two creation narratives (Genesis 1: 27-28 and 5: 1-2),[44] and had interpreted that the first Genesis account included both sexes and referred to an Adam who was an entirely spiritual creature, while, in a noncorporeal way, being both male and female. The second account of an originally male creature out of whom a female one was subsequently created concerned a carnal Adam who is male, and from whom a physical female Eve is made.[45] Philo saw in the two Genesis narratives the creation of two different species of human. There was a 'primal androgyne of no sex and a primal male/ secondary female'.[46] Philo furthermore claimed that only the first, bodiless Adam-creature is in the image of God:

> [H]is male-and-femaleness must be understood spiritually. That is to say that the designation of *this* creature as both male and female means really neither male nor female. This creature is, however, Adam, or at any rate, the Idea of Adam, and therefore while neither male nor female, he is also somehow male. This transcendental androgyne, like Adam himself before there was an Eve, only seems to be both male and female, but 'actually' is singularly male.[47]

The first androgyne human is therefore an ideal male - the apparent absence of gender simply means an absence of the female - and although the first Genesis story includes an androgyne creature without sex but existing as pure spirit, this lack of sex in fact means exclusively male to Philo. Even spirit possesses a (male) gender, it seems.

Interestingly enough, in contrast to Philo's interpretation of the relationship between first and second creation narratives in Genesis is the interpretation of the same textual relationship by the rabbis of late antiquity. 'The dominant rabbinic interpretation insisted on the first male-and-female human as a physical hermaphrodite':[48]

> According to the midrashic interpretation of the early Rabbis, the primordial Adam was a dual-sexed creature in one body. The story in the second chapter of Genesis is the story of the splitting off of the two equal halves of an

[36] Schmitt 1999, 162; Classen 2002, lxix note 176.
[37] Augustine in Bettenson 1984, 661.
[38] *Ibid*, 663.
[39] Salisbury 1996, 82.
[40] Daston and Park 1998, 52.
[41] Plato (190b-192a) in Hamilton 1951, 1974, 59-63.

[42] The interested reader can trace the distribution of Plato's text in medieval manuscripts in the following monograph devoted to the subject: Brockmann 1992.
[43] Philo: *On the Creation* 1.24 and *Allegorical Interpretation of Genesis* II in Colson and Whitaker 1929, 227 paragraph 4, and Tertullian: 'Septim Florens', *Liber adversus Valentin*, chp. 33.
[44] In Boyarin's (Boyarin 2003, 4) translation from the Hebrew these read: 'And God created the earth-creature in his image; in the image of God, He created him; male and female He created them. And God blessed them, and God said to them: Reproduce and fill the earth' (Gen. 1: 27-28). 'This is the book of the Generation of Adam, on the day that God created Adam in the image of God he made him. Male and female he created them, and he blessed them, and called their name Adam, on the day he created them' (Gen. 5: 1-2).
[45] Boyarin 2003, 5.
[46] *Ibid*, 5.
[47] *Ibid*.
[48] *Ibid*, 26.

originary body.[49]

Reminiscent of the explanation given by Aristophanes in Plato's *Symposium* and in Jewish thought, we find here the separation of an androgynous pair of joined twins:

> And God said let us make a human ... R. Samuel the son of Nahman said: When the Holiness (Be it blessed) created the first human, He made it two-faced, then He sawed it and made a back for this one and a back for that one. They objected to him: but it says, 'He took one of his ribs (sela[c]).' He answered [it means], 'one of his sides', similarly to that which is written, 'And the side (sela[c]) of the tabernacle' [Exodus 26: 20].[50]

The theme of the primordial androgyne is also touched on in a text by Augustine (*De genesi ad litteram*, XI 1-32),[51] where Augustine says that before the Fall, Adam and Eve were not ashamed of each other's sight, but only after the Fall did sexual lust exist, implying perhaps a post-lapsarian sexual division. Possibly a miniature depicting a pair of hermaphrodites in the *Livre des merveilles* also relates to this pre-lapsarian notion,[52] following Plato's *Symposium*, of early human beings having been androgynous, as well as depicting a bucolic scene set among the monstrous race of Androgyni/ Hermaphrodites. There are two paths of interpretation for this miniature. Isidore of Seville is also generally positive, where his material on hermaphrodites makes the following matter-of-fact statement:

> Some arise from a mixture of sex, as those which are called Androgunoi or Hermaphroditai. Hermaphrodites are so called because in them both sexes are manifest. Hermes among the Greeks means 'masculine', Aphrodite, 'feminine'. These have the right breast of a man and the left of a woman and, after coitus in turn can both sire and bear children'.[53]

Later on, Scotus Eriugena (*Periphyseon* 2.532D-533A) speculated that the first man only suffered the division of his nature into male and female as punishment for his disobedience. So in a pre-lapsarian state, humanity was bisexual. And at *Periphyseon* 2.538A, Christ is described as perfect because in him there is neither male nor female. One may compare such sentiments of Eriugena with the biblical passage in Galatians 3: 28, which was originally composed with regard to anti-discrimination: 'There is neither Jew nor Greek, there is neither bond nor free, there is neither male nor female: for ye are all one in Christ Jesus'. In the 14th century, Boccaccio (*Genealogie deorum gentilium libri*) interpreted the tale of Hermaphroditus in Ovid's *Metamorphoses* in such a fashion that: 'dual sexuality represented concord and mutually beneficial influences',[54] where Greeks and barbarians meet culturally at Halicarnassus. Pierre Bersuire (died 1362) provided a Christian interpretation of the same Ovidian Hermaphroditus tale, whereby Christ was seen in Hermaphroditus and humanity in the nymph with whom he joined.[55] And Antonio Beccadelli (1394-1471), going under the pen-name Panormita, used antique literary references to write a provocative and humorous text on hermaphrodites and same-sex relations, the *Hermaphroditus*, dedicated to Cosimo de' Medici.[56] Finally, the alchemical hermaphrodite is 'invested with significant positive value',[57] signifying the male and female principles of the universe by combining sun and moon, earth and water, or man and woman.

The causes of hermaphroditism

With alchemy being at the juncture of philosophy and natural science, this brings us thematically onto medieval biological ideas surrounding hermaphroditism. There were two competing theories as to the natural causes for hermaphrodites. One theory posited biological explanations in a symmetrical or scaled schema: according to this, male and female are two endpoints on a spectrum (such as left and right position of the foetus in the womb), but hermaphrodites fall midway in the spectrum: the medical idea of the seven-celled uterus.[58] This tradition on the cause of hermaphrodites apparently 'viewed hermaphrodites as truly intermediate in sex, neither male nor female, but exactly in between'.[59] According to notions deriving from Hippocrates and Galen - by way of Byzantine systematization and a widely-disseminated 12th-century treatise *De spermate* -[60] the human uterus had two cavities, with three warmer divisions on the right cavity engendering males, three colder ones on the left engendering females, and a 7th in the middle responsible for producing hermaphrodites.[61] Giles of Rome, in *De formatione corporis humani in utero*, writing c. 1276, mentions various causes of hermaphroditism relating to general principles and secondary causes such as diet, climate, and heavenly influences, but rejects the secondary causes in favour of principal ones as alone sufficient for the 'occasional appearance of hermaphroditism'.[62] A treatise from the second half of the 12th century, *Anatomia magistri Nicolai phisici*, had also described a seven-celled uterus.[63] Many more medieval medical and natural-philosophical texts referred to a seven-celled uterus.[64] A combination of the idea of the dominant seed and the ensuing foetal position in the maternal uterus is found in a collection of 12th-century medical texts known as

---

49 *Ibid*, 27.

50 Cited in Boyarin 2003, 27, cf. Jehuda and Albeck (eds) 1965, 54-5.

51 Corpus Scriptorum Ecclesiasticorum Latinorum (1866-): 28, 1, published Vienna: F. Tempsky.

52 Paris, Bibliothèque nationale, MS Fr. 2810. fol. 195v.

53 Isidore of Seville in Sharpe 1964: 52, *Etymology*, in the section on monsters at part 3, chp. 11.38ff. Isidore draws on Pliny, *Natural History* 8.2 and 11.49, and on Augustine, *The City of God* 16.8.

54 Rubin 1994, 107 and note 42.

55 cf. Rubin 1994, 107 and note 43.

56 Hergemöller 1992, 22 and note 29 for list of modern editions of Beccadelli's works.

57 Cadden 1993, 209.

58 Bynum 1992, 221, f. Bynum 1992, 384-5 notes 109 and 110 for further bibliographical references.

59 Daston and Park 1996, 119.

60 Pahta 1998, 94-8 for textual transmission, 173 for reference to seven-celled uterus. Today some 38 Latin manuscripts survive, ranging in date from the 12th to the 15th century, held by libraries in England, France, Germany, Italy, Switzerland and the Vatican, which appears to indicate the text's former wide distribution; two of the manuscripts now in England are associated with named owners or copyists: Hermann Zurke of Greifswald, personal physician to Humphrey, Duke of Gloucester, copied one in 1451, and another is associated with Roger Marchall, royal physician to Edward IV.

61 Siraisi 1990, 91-6.

62 Hewson 1975, 186.

63 cf. Rubin 1994, 103 notes 11 and 12; 104 note 13 on the anatomy of Mondino de' Liuzzi.

64 Cf. bibliography provided by Cadden 1993, 93.

the *Prose Salernitan Questions*.[65] Michael Scot (active c. 1200-35), in his *Phisionomia* addressed to emperor Frederick II, discussed human generation, and in that context linked the seven planets with the formation of the child in the womb. Drawing on the seven-celled uterus theory, he postulated that a woman could bear as many as seven children simultaneously (septuplets) because of the availability of seven uterine cells. In such a case a 'child conceived in the middle one of the seven cells of the matrix will be a hermaphrodite'.[66]

An astrological riddle in the form of a poem attributed to the 12th-century archbishop Hildebert of Tours had touched on celestial influence over the developing foetus, whereby Phoebus was linked to a boy, Mars to a girl, but Juno was neither one nor the other:

> While my pregnant mother bore me in the womb, 'tis said the gods deliberated what she should bring forth. Phoebus said, 'It is a boy'; Mars, 'A girl'; Juno, 'Neither'. So when I was born, I was a hermaphrodite. When I seek to die, the goddess says, 'He shall be slain by a weapon'; Mars, 'By crucifixion'; Phoebus, 'By drowning'. So it turned out. A tree shades the water; I climb it; the sword I carry by chance slips from its scabbard; I myself fall upon it; my trunk is impaled in the branches; my head falls into the river. Thus I, man, woman, and neither, suffered flood, sword, and cross.[67]

The poem is meant to represent the fulfillment of a horoscope. It exists in another version, far longer, by Peter Riga, entitled *De ortu et morte pueri monstruosi*; and Matthew of Vendôme mentioned a poem *Hic et haec hermaphroditus homo* among a list of his own works. One may also mention here a physiognomic text by Guilhelmus de Mirica, the *Physionomia*, dealing with the generation of hermaphrodites, manlike women and womanly men.[68] According to the *Reductiorum phisonomie* of Rolandus Scriptoris, written about 1430 and dedicated to the duke of Bedford, a relatively low level of bodily hair was characteristic of women, eunuchs, northern people, and melancholic people,[69] although hermaphrodites are not explicitly mentioned in this text, presumably subsumed under the stereotype of eunuchs and/or effeminate men.

Further anatomical evidence comes from a medical text, *Sapientia artis medicinae*, which lists the number of bones in the human body; men possess a total of 228 bones, women only possess 226, but a people called the Frigisci possess 227. According to Klaus-Dietrich Fischer, the term *Frigisci* refers to the Phrygians, that is a people of Asia Minor from among whom the priests of Cybele were recruited, notorious for castrating themselves in the service of the goddess,[70] and as self-created eunuchs therefore occupied that ambiguous territory between male and female also inhabited by sodomites and hermaphrodites.

Besides multi-celled uteri and divergent numbers of bones, the origin of sperm in the left or right testicle was also thought to influence the gender characteristics of the ensuing conception. According to the *Liber de coitu* of Constantinus Africanus (1015 - before 1099), which survives in at least 22 Latin manuscripts, as well as in a 15th-century partial translation into Middle English,[71] when sperm which had originated in the left testicle falls onto the right part of the uterus, the result is a masculine or manly woman, and when sperm from the right testicle falls onto the left part of the uterus, then an effeminate man will be the outcome; except that almighty God can at all times grant to whom he will to engender a male and to whom he will a female as He only knows:

> Forsoth, sum leches han seid if seede the whiche goeth bifore of the lift partie [of the testicles] fal on the right partie of the matrice, than it makith a womman masculyne or manly; and if to that whiche issueth of the right side fallith in the lift partie of the matrice, makyth a man effemynat, save this: as myghty is God to graunte to whom he wil to gendre a male and to whom he wil a femal, as he knowith.[72]

Although the presence of the middle uterine chamber and other anatomical models might lead one to believe that a hermaphrodite is a natural being, and therefore a third sex, this interpretation needs to be balanced by the persistent medieval attempts to squeeze hermaphrodites into one or the other of the two sexes, into either male or female roles.

The other theory of the origin of hermaphrodites centred around the degeneration of sperm at the moment of procreation and the negative influence of female menses.[73] According to this high medieval scholastic theory - which, having re-discovered Aristotle,[74] posits a hierarchical order of possible outcomes of the moment of fertilisation: at best, a male child will result, then a female child, then a monster, then nothing at all - this is an example of the philosophical *horror vacui*, which stems from the notion that nature abhors a vacuum. The degenerative theory of the aetiology of hermaphroditism could be expanded on, however, and the condition of hermaphrodites medicalized even further. For example, Albertus Magnus in the mid-13th century produced an influential medieval scientific explanation for hermaphroditism, by embracing and adding to Aristotelian theories.[75] Accordingly, hermaphroditism was perceived to be caused by an accident of nature, similar to that which could produce growths such as tumours; but underlying whatever secondary sexual characteristics a hermaphrodite might have there was the true sex and the primary sexual organs.[76] Already according to Aristotle, the sex of hermaphrodites was 'never more than apparently ambiguous, since the sex of the whole foetus was determined by the heat of the heart, which in turn determined the complexion of the body as a whole'.[77] Here

[65] Lawn 1979, 103, text B, 193; English translation in Cadden 1993, 201.
[66] Thorndike 1923, 329. Thorndike is referring to Michael Scot's *Phisionomia*, edition of 1740, cap. 7, 227.
[67] Thorndike 1923, 109; cf. Migne 1857-1939: vol. 171, col. 1446.
[68] Cadden 1993, 202.
[69] Ziegler 2005, 514; the manuscript is in Lisbon, Biblioteca Ajuda, ms. 52.XIII.18, fol. 49r.
[70] Fischer 1985, 262.
[71] Matheson 2006, 287-93.
[72] *Ibid*, 307.
[73] cf. Wood 1981 on medieval attitude toward menses.
[74] Aristotle, *On the Generation of Animals*, bk. 4 chp 1 and chp. 4.
[75] cf. Rubin 1994, 102 note 10.
[76] Cadden 1993, 212.
[77] Daston and Park 1996, 119. Daston and Park are referring to Aristotle, *On the Generation of Animals*, bk. 4 chp. 1.

is clear evidence that instead of treating hermaphroditism as some kind of third sex, or even intersex as modern expression does, medieval biological science thought of hermaphrodites as deformed, damaged or corrupted males or females, but males or females nevertheless and not something in between - hence medieval notions placed hermaphrodites very much into the established duality of the sexes and of gender roles. However, Albertus Magnus questioned Aristotle's categorical statement that one could always know the true sex of the hermaphrodite from their complexion by pointing out:

> However, sometimes even the complexion of the heart is so intermediate that it is scarcely possible to discern which of the sexes should prevail.
>
> (*tamen aliquando etiam complexio cordis ita media est quod vix discerni potest quis sexuum praevaleat*).[78]

But having identified such deviations from the norm, immediate attempts were made to suppress them, by reducing them to: 'permutations of the conventional categories of masculine and feminine'.[79]

Hermaphroditism and disability

Having glanced at medieval biological and medical causes of hermaphroditism, it is perhaps apposite for us to consider to what extent a hermaphrodite might be regarded as disabled, both by medieval and modern society. This line of thought immediately throws up the problem of what is actually meant by the category disabled, especially the problem of what does it mean in modern 21st century society, and what may disability have meant in a medieval context? The most fruitful approach, still, is to employ the social model of disability. This makes a distinction between impairment in a medical sense (which relates to loss of a function at an organic, anatomical, biological level), and disability as the social or cultural construct superimposed upon that impairment.[80] So while a modern hermaphrodite (or intersex person) may be considered anatomically deviant (and, according to the medical profession, in need of corrective surgery) they are not considered disabled in the same way as, say, a wheelchair user or a visually impaired person would be.

But social context is all. While the biological otherness of the hermaphrodite may not intrinsically be enough to render them disabled, the arguments for curtailment or downright negation of social rights or positions based on such a differing biology would do so. One aspect where medieval law, theology, and medical knowledge intersect is in the context of hermaphrodites and procreation. In that sense a hermaphrodite, since without procreative function, could be regarded as impaired. But the ability to procreate is valued differently in different cultures, in that in modern Western society the ability to have children is no longer seen as a perquisite to marriage, and in industrialised societies hermaphroditism is not classified as a disability. However, in many traditional cultures, as anthropologists like to call it, 'being a member of a family and having children are far more important to being a person than work capacity or appearance',[81] and therefore in such a context hermaphroditism can be regarded as disabling. Anthropological research has shown a wide variety of *reactions* to people with impairments across different cultures, and hermaphroditism and intersex are no exceptions. In some cultures people with ambiguous genitalia are killed at birth (among the Chagga of eastern Africa/ Tanzania) while in other cultures the birth of a hermaphrodite child was considered to be a fortunate event, for example among the Navaho Indians.[82] Cross-cultural comparisons provide valuable insights into how societies other than our own react to and deal with phenomena beyond the normal range of quotidian experience.

The fact that medieval law became involved with issues of which sex a person was to have indicates to me that in the middle ages hermaphrodites were seen as disabled (by virtue of their sterility, with perhaps the social consequence being no right to marry), but a hermaphrodite was nevertheless part of God's created universe. There are sound biological reasons why hermaphrodites exist, which the natural philosophers tried to understand and explain to the level of scientific knowledge and standards of their time. Ecclesiastical authors, on the other hand, became concerned about the inability of hermaphrodites to consummate marriage. Therefore hermaphrodites had to be: 'directed, through education and socialisation, into one social and sexual category or another. They had to behave and be recognised either as men or as women, an identity that once chosen must be adhered to'.[83]

The ability of married couples to have sexual relations gained legal importance, in canon law that is, during the 8th and 9th centuries.[84] Hence the hermaphrodite had to be definitive in his or her choice of gender, if not sex, since such a choice would impact on the ability or permission to marry. Peter the Chanter in the late 12th century, in his *Verbum abbreviatum*, stated that God may allow the birth of an androgynous foetus which, with regard to the future generative act, is 'not exclusively masculine or feminine, but with instruments for both acting and receiving'.[85] The church grants such individuals the right to choose the sex 'which is best aroused and to marry accordingly':.

> The Lord formed man from the slime of the earth on the plain of Damascus, later fashioning woman from his rib in Eden. Thus in considering the formation of woman, lest any should believe they would be hermaphrodites, he stated, "Male and female created he them", as if to say, "There will not be intercourse of men with men or women with women, but only of men with women and vice versa". For this reason the church allows a hermaphrodite - that is, someone with the organs of both sexes, capable of either active or passive functions - to use the organ by which (s)he is most aroused or the one to which (s)he is more susceptible. If (s)he is more active [literally, "lustful"], (s)he may wed as a man, but if (s)he is more passive, (s)he may

[78] Albertus Magnus in Stadler 1916, 1920, 1225; cf. Cadden 1993, 212.
[79] Cadden 1993, 212.
[80] Metzler 2006, 20-1.
[81] Ingstad and White 1995, 11.
[82] Neubert and Cloerkes 1994, 42-4.
[83] Hadley 2001, 185.
[84] Brundage 1987, 144.
[85] Baldwin 1994, 45.

marry as a woman. If, however, (s)he should fail with one organ, the use of the other can never be permitted, but (s) he must be perpetually celibate to avoid any similarity to the role inversion of sodomy, which is detested by God'.

(*Item. Isti qui hoc laborant vicio androgei fiunt nunc agentes nunc pacientes. Quia utrumque usurpant officium quia habentes orificium. Quod ne liceret cum dominus virum plasmasset de limo terre in agro damasceno, formaturus mulierem de costa eius in paradiso? Ne crederet eos quis androgeos preocupans formationem mulieris ait* [Genesis 1:27]: *masculum et feminam creavit eos quasi non erat consortium viri ad virum vel mulieris ad mulierem sed tantum viri ad mulierem et converso. Item. Propter ignominiam istam quam inferunt creatori et nature permittit dominus fetus nasci corruptos et androgeos qui nec plene viri nec plene femine sunt. Unde ecclesia homini androgeo, id est, habenti instrumentum utriusque sexus aptum, scilicet, ad agendum et paciendum, optionem eligendi indulget in quo velit sexu permanere. Quo vero instrumento magis calescit, quove magis est infirmus, permittit ei uti. Si magis calescit ut vir, permittit eum ducere. Si vero calescit magis ut mulier permittit eum nubere. Si autem in illo instrumento defecerit, numquam conceditur ei usus reliqui sed perpetuo continebit ut sic vicium illud extirpetur. Et nulla tenus agentis et pacientis officium sequens vestigia alternitatis vicii sodomitici a deo detestabilis posse convenire uni et eidem persone credatur*).[86]

Peter the Chanter also re-emphasised, in his preliminary discussion of Genesis 1:27, that men and women are distinct from one another; not one but two people were created, nor were they of a single sex but created as two and not as androgynes, that is, not as hermaphrodites who possess the genitalia of both men and women:

because God created man not only as one man but two, not in one sex only but on both sides because as male and female he created them not androgynes, that is, not as hermaphrodites who simultaneously have the instruments of men and women.

(*quod deus creavit hominem non solum unum hominem sed duos, nec in uno tantum sexu sed in utroque quia masculum et feminam creavit eos non androgeos, id est, non ermafroditos qui viri et mulieris simul habent instrumentum*).[87]

The theological problem of hermaphroditism is further explored by Robert of Courson, one time pupil of Peter, in his *Summa* XLII, 18, who engaged himself with the problem that in the hermaphrodite the two sexes cannot be contingent and flourish equally, therefore one sex must always prevail, and the emergence during puberty of the 'stronger' sex will decide the outcome:

The solution that the physicians have transmitted is that it cannot be contingent that the two sexes in the hermpahrodite flourish evenly. In reality it is necessary that always one obtains the privilege ... because as the human law says always in such things the sex by age enflamed decides.

(*Solutio ut tradunt phisici non potest contingere quod duo sexus in ermafrodito equaliter vigeant. Immo oportet quod semper unus obtineat privilegium ... quia ut dicit lex humana semper sexus incalescentis etatis preiudicat in talibus*).[88]

After hermaphrodites have chosen their gender, they may never change their roles but must remain acting out the chosen one, according to Peter.[89] Perhaps this is the reason why hermaphrodites, even if identified as such at birth, could wait until the age of majority to make the final decision on their gender: it was important to get it right, so to speak, and anatomical manifestations in a newborn baby could change, grow, or diminish over time during the physiological development to adulthood, hence it was a good idea to wait until then. 'The whole theory of marriage was challenged by the hermaphrodite, who could fulfil the requirement for consent, while retaining ambiguity or lacking the ability to have fruitful intercourse'.[90] Medieval Islamic societies, by contrast, did not suffer from the same pervasive fear of homosexuality as medieval Christian ones, and permitted hermaphrodites to marry,[91] providing, of course, a gender had been assigned juridically to such a person.

The western medieval notion of choice, never mind a choice at age of maturity, contrasts startlingly with the modern medical viewpoint of intersex. Intersexed bodies in modern industrialised societies are often tidied away soon after birth through corrective surgery in an attempt to normalise them. This not infrequently has negative physical and psychological side-effects for the people concerned, from feelings of violation and powerlessness, to the wider question of inferiority against the perceived normal body.[92] The topic is brilliantly explored in a novel by Jeffrey Eugenides, *Middlesex* (2002).

Conclusions

Medieval hermaphrodites and intersex people - generally - escaped the snipping and cutting, if not to say mutilation, of modern surgery. The writings of the medical profession in the middle ages were 'content with quoting some anecdote, or with pointing out, as does Avicenna, that certain hermaphrodites may, as they prefer, be either a man or a woman: the Church forced them to choose'.[93] Quoting Avicenna and Albucasis,[94] Guy de Chauliac in his *Chirurgia* mentions that there is a surgical procedure for removing penis and testicles found above the vulva in otherwise female bodies ('cured by cutting'):

[86] English translation given by Boswell 1980, 375-6: Peter the Chanter: *Verbum abbreviatum* (long version). MS Vatican, Reg. lat. 106, fols. 153rb-154va, cited in Baldwin 1994, 248.

[87] Peter the Chanter: Paris, Arsenal, MS 44, p. 7a, and London, British Library, MS Royal 2C8, fol. 4va, cited in Baldwin 1994, 45 note 6.

[88] Baldwin 1994, 45 note 6: Paris, Bibliothèque nationale, MS lat. 14524, fol. 144va.

[89] Baldwin 1994, 45.

[90] Rubin 1994, 105.

[91] Sanders 1991, 88.

[92] Cornwall 2006. Modern comparisons, like my cross-cultural comparisons above, have value for the same reasons: permitting different viewpoints re: the unfamiliar, and pointing out the social construction of viewpoints, just as disability is a social construct.

[93] Jacquart and Thomasset 1988, 141.

[94] Details of the passages are given by Rubin 1994, 102 notes 5 and 6 respectively.

> Hermafrodicia is the nature of double kynde. And it is in men (after Albucasis) after two maneres, for sometyme it is in the place that is apperynge under the stones. In a womman forsothe there is another in the whiche a yerde [penis] and prive stones [testicles] apperen above the prive chose [vulva]. And thai ben ofte tymes cured by kyttynge, as Avicen saith, but noght that forsothe that maketh water, as Albucasis saith.[95]

Theoretically this sounds promising from a medical viewpoint, but in the context of the overall abilities of medieval surgery, it is doubtful to what extent this operation was carried out.[96] There is, however, mention of one allegedly successful surgical operation in a chronicle made in 1308-14 by the Dominicans of Colmar, in Alsace. This chronicle recorded for the year 1300 the case of a wife who had passed as a proper woman for ten years, but had been unable to consummate her marriage, which was dissolved. On her way to Rome (perhaps on hopeful pilgrimage during the jubilee year), she stopped at Bologna, where a surgeon cut open her vagina to reveal a penis and testicles hidden beneath or inside. On her return home she led a life as a true and *real* man, even able to perform hard physical work:[97]

> In a town near Bern ... a woman lived for ten years with a man. Since she could not have sex with a man she was separated [from her partner] by the spiritual court. In Bologna (on her way to Rome), her vagina was cut open by a surgeon, and a penis and testicles came out. She returned home, married a wife, did hard [physical] labour, and had proper and adequate sexual congress with her wife.[98]

Here is perhaps the only medieval case of an allegedly successful operation.

Returning back to where we started from, the law. Medical professionals were mainly content with testifying in court cases as to the ability or inability of a person to fulfil their conjugal debt, as in a case in 1331 at Perelada in northeastern Catalonia. A man named Guillem Castelló wanted to prove to the court that his wife Berengaria 'could not fulfil her conjugal debt nor conceive nor bear a child' and called in a surgeon, who in the presence of a matron of the town 'raised the knees of the said Berengaria and examined [her]'.[99] The surgeon declared under oath his assessment was, basically, that Berengaria was more male than female:

> [S]he has a male penis and testicles like a man; and is so narrow that she can barely urinate through an opening that she has in a fissure that she has in the vulva, [a fissure] that lies beneath her penis; and has a flap stretched between her thighs like the wings of a bat, which covers the fissure in the vulva whenever she draws her knees toward her head; and she has more the aspect of a man than a woman, and there is no way in which Guillem or any other man can lie with her.
>
> (*Qui quidem medicus supradictus ad instanciam dicti Guillelmi vocavit dictam Berengariam una cum domina Cotona filia Guillelmi Bartholomei quondam de Castilione et in presencia dicte domine Cotone elevavit genua dicte Berengarie et recognovit et inspexit si ea que dicta erant et requisita per dictum Guillelmus erant vera quibus siquidem supradictam inspectis et recognitis per dictum medicum idem medicus dixit virtute iuramenti per eum prestiti in posse curie ville Perelate in principio sui regiminis quod dicta Berengaria habebat virgam virilem et testiculos ad modum hominis et est arta ita quod vix potest mingere per quoddam foramen parvum quod habet in fissura vulve quam habet suptus dictam virgam virilem et habet pellem inter crura sua stensam ad modum alarum vespertilionis que cohoperit fissuram dicte vulve tociens quociens ipsa Berengaria vertit genua sua versus faciem suam et quod habet formam virilem plus quam muliebrem, its quod dictus Guillelmus nec alter homo posse iacere secum nec habere rem carnaliter nec ipsa posset reddere ullatenus debitum coniugalis nec concipere nec infantare*).[100]

The anatomical description was comprehensible enough for a modern medical professional, Dr Peter English of Duke University, to diagnose that Berengaria was 'probably a biological male with third-degree hypospadias'.[101] Nevertheless, one could argue that medieval medical approaches to hermaphroditism had a lot in common with medical approaches of that period toward physical impairment: both 'conditions' were untreatable and incurable by the then-available medical means (and to an extent are still so today), so that, in general, medieval medical discourse was content with describing the symptoms, theorizing about aetiology and philosophizing about possible meanings.

In conclusion, hermaphroditism was looked upon as an impairment in the medieval period, in the sense that it was an incurable, permanent, physical aberration from the anatomical norm which excluded the affected individual from certain aspects of *normal* social life, such as marriage and procreation. The aspect of exclusion also meant that one could regard medieval hermaphrodites as *disabled* in the modern sense. Similar to other modern disabilities, there are material and social methods of trying to alleviate the disability. The choice of sex and corresponding gender role of medieval hermaphrodites was to them such a social method of alleviation, a prop, in an attempt to overcome a socially and culturally perceived disability, much as a crutch enabled mobility in a cripple. But methods to alleviate disability, such as a wheelchair, can also be forms of taming, by turning a concrete and individually-experienced disability into the abstract and symbolic, in that the sexless figure on the wheelchair, a ubiquitous part of modern signage in public spaces, becomes the symbol for *all* disability. Hence the medieval hermaphrodite's choice

[95] Guy de Chauliac in Ogden 1971, 529.
[96] Translation in Rubin 1994, 101; Jacquart and Thomasset 1988, 141.
[97] Rubin 1994, 101.
[98] Citing Scriptores 17, 1828, 225. For contextualisation of this chronicle, as part of a new direction in medieval historiography, moving away from the *gesta*, the great deeds of the powerful, toward a kind of social history with localized focus, cf. Kleinschmidt 1972.
99 McVaugh 1993, 206.

[100] McVaugh 1993, 206, citing the record in the archives of Gerona (Spain), Arxiu Històric Provincial, fons de Perelada, manual de Bernat Sunyer 26 bis/52v (24 August 1331).
[101] McVaugh 1993, 206.

becomes normalization, alleviation and oppression all at the same time, through reinforcement of societal norms.

Lastly, one must not forget that the topic of medieval hermaphroditism is primarily one of philological reconstruction, reflecting the medieval authors' own reconstruction and reworking of earlier (classical Greek and Latin) texts. The medieval hermaphrodite can mainly be a signifier, an emblematic character, or even the product of a philosophical thought-game, but rarely a real, flesh-and-blood person. True hermaphroditism - as opposed to individual genital variation - is nowadays a very rare biological occurrence, and there is no reason to suppose that the ratio of this congenital abnormality would have been different in the past, or that genetic mutations operated very much differently among what were after all anatomically modern humans. For the middle ages we cannot, of course, obtain the sort of statistical detail for occurrences of hermaphroditism per 1000 of the population that we have available for modern western society. Hypospadias, for example, the condition that Berengaria may have had, occurs in about 1 in 300 boys to a greater or lesser degree, but is usually surgically modified before the age of two in modern Great Britain.[102]

We can not even look for incidences of hermaphrodites in medieval burials, since, as a purely soft-tissue manifestation, hermaphroditism is invisible archaeologically. For all we know, there may have been more cases of medieval hermaphrodites than the three that surface in the literature: the unnamed female hermaphrodite in the Alsace mentioned in the Colmar chronicle for 1281, the wife in the same chronicle of 1300, and Berengaria from Catalonia in 1331 - interestingly enough all these were hermaphrodites with greater *female* genital characteristics who misbehave by trying to act male, or who are really males hidden inside female bodies. One may possibly add as a fourth the case of the Venetian Rolandino/Rolandina in 1354, where the reverse (female inside a male) situation occurred, at least in behavioural terms.

The interesting question therefore is: were there really no more instances of hermaphroditism for the entire middle ages, or was it rather an oversight or a case of non-recognition by the intellectual authors, the natural historians, philosopher-theologians and medical writers? If we assume that the ratio of congenital abnormality was the same for the medieval period as nowadays, it seems unlikely that there were fewer hermaphrodites then than in the present. Instead, one must assume that the learned writers were more interested in philosophical (and even philological) musings, following in the footsteps of one classical authority or another, than real-life observations. Intellectuals like Albertus Magnus, who allegedly interrogated the fishwives at their market stalls to gain insights into specific female questions, seem to have been the exception. Had more medieval writers left their cloister or their university lodgings and spoken to the *rustici*, the great unwashed, uneducated, uncultured mass of the peasantry, they might have come across more instances of medieval hermaphroditism. For the peasants, who surely would periodically have encountered all sorts of strange, weird and wonderful abnormalities in the domestic animals around them, similar abnormalities in humans may well have just been considered part and parcel of life and not something to get particularly excited about.

[102] Smith 2000, 870.

Bibliography

Baldwin, J.W. 1994. *The Language of Sex: Five Voices from Northern France around 1200*, Chicago and London: University of Chicago Press.

Bettenson. H. (trans.) 1984. *Augustine, The City of God*, London: Penguin.

Bildhauer, B. and Mills, R. 2003. 'Introduction: Conceptualizing the Monstrous,' in B. Bildhauer and R. Mills (eds), *The Monstrous Middle Ages*, 1-27, Cardiff: University of Wales Press.

Boswell, J. 1980. *Christianity, Social Tolerance, and Homosexuality*, Chicago and London: University of Chicago Press.

Boyarin, D. 2003. 'On the History of the Early Phallus,' in S. Farmer and C. B. Pasternak (eds), *Gender and Difference in the Middle Ages* (Medieval Cultures vol. 32), 3-44, Minneapolis: University of Minnesota Press.

Brisson, L. 2002. *Sexual Ambivalence: Androgyny and Hermaphroditism in Graeco-Roman Antiquity*, Los Angeles: California University Press.

Brockmann, C. 1992. *Die handschriftliche Überlieferung von Platons Symposium*. Serta Graeca. Beiträge zur Erforschung griechischer Texte, Bd. 2, Wiesbaden: Dr. Ludwig Reichert Verlag.

Brundage, J.A. 1987. *Law, Sex, and Christian Society in Medieval Europe*, Chicago and London: University of Chicago Press.

Bynum, C.W. 1992. *Fragmentation and Redemption: Essays on Gender and the Human Body in Medieval Religion*, New York: Zone Books.

Cadden, J. 1993. *Meanings of Sex Difference in the Middle Ages: Medicine, Science, and Culture*, Cambridge: Cambridge University Press.

Cadden, J. 1996. 'Western Medicine and Natural Philosophy', in V.L. Bullough and J.A. Brundage (eds), *Handbook of Medieval Sexuality*, 51-80, New York and London: Garland.

Cadden, J. 1997. 'Sciences/Silences: The Natures and Languages of "Sodomy" in Peter of Abano's *Problemata* Commentary', in K. Lochrie, P. McCracken and J.A. Schultz (eds), *Constructing Medieval Sexuality*, 40-57, Minneapolis: University of Minnesota Press.

Classen, A. 2002. *Meeting the Foreign in the Middle Ages*, New York and London: Routledge.

Colson F. H. and Whitaker G. H. (transl.) 1929. 'Allegorical Interpretation of Genesis II', *Philo in Ten Volumes*, vol. I, Cambridge, MA: Loeb Classical Library.

Cornwall, S. 2006. 'Some Resonances between Intersex Conditions and the Theology of Disability', paper given at Eleventh Joint Postgraduate Conference, 11 March 2006, Bath Spa University.

Damme, C. 1978. 'Infanticide: The worth of an infant under law', *Medical History*, **22/1,** 1-24.

Daston, L. and Park K. 1985. 'Hermaphrodites in Renaissance France', *Critical Matrix*, **1/5**, 1-19.

Daston, L. and Park K. 1996. 'The Hermaphrodite and the Orders of Nature: Sexual Ambiguity in Early Modern France', in L. Fradenburg and C. Freccero (eds), *Premodern Sexualities*, 117-36, London and New York: Routledge.

Daston, L. and Park K. 1998. *Wonders and the Order of Nature 1150-1750*, New York: Zone Books.

Eugenides, J. 2002. *Middlesex*, London: Bloomsbury.

Fischer, K.-D. 1985. 'Ein weiteres spätantikes Zeugnis für die Zahnzahl der Eunuchen', *Medizinhistorisches Journal*, **20/3**, 261-2.

Foucault, M. 1998. *Über Hermaphrodismus. Der Fall Barbin* (published as *Herculine Barbin dite Alexina B., presente par Michel Foucault*, Paris, 1978), transl. and ed. W. Schäffner and J. Vogl, Edition Suhrkamp Neue Folge 733, Frankfurt-a-M: Suhrkamp.

Garton, S. 2004. *Histories of Sexuality: Antiquity to Sexual Revolution*, London: Equinox.

Green, M. 2000. *Women's Healthcare in the Medieval West: Texts and Contexts*, Aldershot: Ashgate Variorum.

Hadley, D. M. 2001. 'Fear and fantasy: sexuality and medieval societies', in L. Bevan (ed.), *Indecent Exposure: Sexuality, Society and the Archaeological Record*, 179-200, Glasgow: Cruithne Press.

Hamilton, W. transl. 1951, 1974. *Plato: The Symposium*, London: Penguin.

Hassig, D. 1995. *Medieval Bestiaries: Text, Image, Ideology*, Cambridge: Cambridge University Press.

Hergemöller, B.-U. 1992. 'Grundfragen zum Verständnis gleichgeschlechtlichen Verhaltens im späten Mittelalter', in R. Lautmann and A. Taeger (eds), *Männerliebe im alten Deutschland. Sozialgeschichtliche Abhandlungen*, 9-38, Berlin: Verlag rosa Winkel.

Hewson, M.A. 1975. *Giles of Rome and the Medieval Theory of Conception: a Study of the De formatione corporis humane in utero*, London: Athlone Press.

Ingstad, B. and White, S.R. (eds) 1995. *Disability and Culture*, Berkeley - Los Angeles - London: University of California Press.

Jacquart, D. and Thomasset, C. 1988. *Sexuality and Medicine in the Middle Ages*, transl. M. Adamso. Cambridge: Polity Press.

Jehuda, T. and Albeck, H. (eds) 1965. *Genesis Rabbah*, Jerusalem.

Karras, R. M. 2005. *Sexuality in Medieval Europe: Doing unto others*, New York and London: Routledge.

Kleinschmidt, E. 1972. 'Die Colmarer Dominikaner-Geschichtsschreibung im 13. und 14. Jahrhundert', *Deutsches Archiv für Erforschung des Mittelalters*, **28**, 371–438.

Krüger, P. (ed.) 1971. *Corpus iuris civilis: Institutiones, Digesta*, 21st edn, Dublin and Zurich: Weidmann.

Kuefler, M. S. 1996. 'Castration and Eunuchism in the Middle Ages', in V. L. Bullough and J. A. Brundage (eds), *Handbook of Medieval Sexuality*, 279-306, New York and London: Garland.

Lawn, B. 1979. *The Prose Salernitan Questions* (Auctores Britannici Medii Aevi V), London: British Academy/ Oxford University Press.

McCarthy C. 2004. 'The Plaint of Nature', in C. McCarthy (ed.), *Love, Sex and Marriage in the Middle Ages: A Sourcebook*, 177-9, London and New York: Routledge.

McVaugh, M. R. 1993. *Medicine Before the Plague*, Cambridge: Cambridge University Press.

Matheson, L. M. 2006. 'Constantinus Africanus: De coitu', in M.T. Tavormina (ed.), *Sex, Aging, and Death in a Medieval Medical Compendium: Trinity College Cambridge MS R.14.52, its Texts, Language, and Scribe*, 287-326, Tempe, Arizona: Arizona Center for Medieval and Renaissance Studies.

Metzler, I. 2006. *Disability in Medieval Europe: Thinking about physical impairment during the high Middle Ages, c. 1100-1400*, London and New York: Routledge.

Migne, J. P. (ed.) 1857-1939. *Patrologia Latina*, 161 volumes, Paris: Garnier.

Neubert, D. and Cloerkes, G. 1994. *Behinderung und Behinderte in verschiedenen Kulturen. Eine vergleichende Analyse ethnologischer Studien*, Heidelberg: Edition Schindele.

Ogden M.S. (ed.) 1971. *The Cyrurgie of Guy de Chauliac*, Early English Text Society 265, Oxford: Oxford University Press.

Pahta, P. 1998. *Medieval Embryology in the Vernacular: The Case of De Spermate*, Helsinki: Société Néophilologique.

Richardson, H. G. and Sayles, G. O. (eds) 1955. *Fleta*, Selden Society, London: Quaritch.

Rubin, M. 1994. 'The person in the form: medieval challenges to bodily "other"', in S. Kay and M. Rubin (eds), *Framing Medieval Bodies*, 100-22, Manchester and New York: Manchester University Press.

Rubin, M. 1996. 'The Body, Whole and Vulnerable, in Fifteenth-Century England', in B. Hanawalt and D. Wallace (eds), *Bodies and Discipline: Intersections of Literature and History in Fifteenth-Century England* (Medieval Cultures Vol. 9), 19-28, Minneapolis: Minnesota University Press.

Saint-Hilaire, Q. de (ed.) 1889. *Oeuvres complètes d'Eustache Deschamps*, VI, ballad 1129, 49-50, Paris.

Salisbury, J. E. 1996. 'Gendered Sexuality', in V. L. Bullough and J. A Brundage (eds), *Handbook of Medieval Sexuality*, 81-102, New York and London: Garland.

Sanders, P. 1991. 'Gendering the Ungendered Body: Hermaphrodites in Medieval Islamic Law', in N. Keddie and B. Baron (eds), *Women in Middle Eastern History*, 74-95, New Haven: Yale University Press.

Schmitt, K. 1999. 'Minne, Monster, Mutationen: Geschlechterkonstruktionen im 'Alexanderroman' Ulrichs von Etzenbach', in A. Robertshaw and G. Wolf (eds), *Natur und Kultur in der deutschen Literatur des Mittelalters*, 151-62. Tübingen: Niemeyer.

Scriptores 17: 1828. *Annales Colmarienses Minores*, Monumenta Germaniae Historica

Sharpe, W. D. (trans) 1964. 'Isidore of Seville: the medical writing', *Transactions of the American Philosophical Society*, **54/2**, 3-75.

Siraisi, N. G. 1990. *Medieval and Early Renaissance Medicine: An Introduction to Knowledge and Practice*, Chicago and London: University of Chicago Press.

Smith, T. (ed.) 2000. *The British Medical Association Complete Family Health Guide*, London: Dorling Kindersley.

Stadler, H. (ed.) 1916, 1920. *De animalibus*, bk. XVIII, tr. ii, ch. 3, § 66. Beiträge zur Geschichte der Philosophie des Mittelalters 15 and 16, Münster: Aschendorf.

Thorndike, L. 1923. *A History of Magic and Experimental Science*, vol. 2, New York and London: Columbia University Press.

Thorne, S. E. and Woodbine G. (ed. and transl.) 1997. *De legibus et consuetudinibus Angliae*, English and Latin, vol. 2. Buffalo: W. S. Hein. Online at http://hlsl5.law.harvard.edu/bracton/index.htm

Williams, D. 1996. *Deformed Discourse: The Function of the Monster in Medieval Thought and Literature*, Exeter: University of Exeter Press.

Wood, C. T. 1981. 'The Doctor's Dilemma: Sin, salvation, and the menstrual cycle in medieval thought', *Speculum,* **56**, 710-27.

Ziegler, J. 2005. 'Skin and Character in Medieval and Early Renaissance Physiognomy', *Micrologus* [La pelle umana. The Human Skin], **13**, 511-35.

Chapter Five

The nadir of Western Medicine? Texts, contexts and practice in Anglo-Saxon England

Sally Crawford

Introduction

Imagine a line on a graph plotting the progress of medical knowledge in the Western world from the Greeks to the early modern period. The peaks would probably coincide with the flowering of Greek and Roman civilization, with another peak when medical knowledge was renewed from the Arabic world in the Middle Ages. In between these peaks would come a deep trough, and at the bottom of that trough, in the middle of the 'Dark Ages', would be Anglo-Saxon England. Here, medical knowledge, fatally damaged, was suffering what has been described in unflattering terms as 'the last stage of a process that has left no legitimate successor, a final pathological disintegration of the great system of Greek medical thought'.[1]

There are a number of reasons why Anglo-Saxon medical knowledge has been rated so harshly. From the 5th to the 7th centuries - from the withdrawal of the Roman Army to the arrival of Christian missionaries from Ireland, Rome and Merovingian Europe - Anglo-Saxon England was dominated by an illiterate society, whose understanding of medicine has to be extrapolated either from sketchy archaeological evidence, or from later sources whose recording of the past was based on oral tradition. Later, literate Anglo-Saxon England has provided us with a number of lucky documentary survivals which represent a small, and not necessarily representative, proportion of the texts which may once have been written. These texts range from translations of Greek and Roman originals, such as *Peri Didaxeon* and *Medicina de Quadrupedibus*, to compilations based on Mediterranean and native knowledge, written in the vernacular, such as *Lacnunga*.[2] Charms and incantations form part of this corpus, and these have bedevilled the reputation of Anglo-Saxon medicine, not least because they have drawn an entirely disproportionate amount of attention. Translations of the charms into modern English, and interpretations of the 'magical' aspects of Anglo-Saxon medicine, abound.[3] By contrast, the first two volumes Bald's *Leechbook*, an important and substantial 10th century medical compendium, which represent a considered, organised and thoughtful compilation of medical lore - in effect, Anglo-Saxon medicine at its best - are still only accessible to the modern reader in a facsimile of the original Old English text, or in the 19th century English translation by the Reverend Oswald Cockayne.[4]

Given the overwhelming emphasis which the magical and ritual elements of Anglo-Saxon medicine have received, it is not surprising that interpreters of this period of medical history have traditionally either dismissed the period as a backwater of superstition, or have acted as apologists for the period.[5] Subsequent reviews of Anglo-Saxon medical practice challenged the belief that medical knowledge in this period was, at best, a confusion of native magical lore, superstition, and misunderstood Mediterranean texts, and have argued for the strength of rational medical practice and knowledge in later Anglo-Saxon England.[6] The re-evaluation of medical expertise in later Anglo-Saxon England has suffered a new reverse, however: Anglo-Saxon remedies tested in laboratory conditions indicate that, while levels of training amongst Anglo-Saxon doctors may have been high, medical practice ensured that even anti-microbial ingredients, when processed according to the given instructions, would have been rendered ineffective.[7]

What the latest experiments on Anglo-Saxon medical remedies re-iterate is that, in order to successfully gather the ingredients and to prepare and store the mixtures for the prescribed length of time before applying them to the patient, the users of Bald's *Leechbook*, for example, would have had to have been practitioners, rather than lay people hoping to self-medicate. The Anglo-Saxon doctor, the experimenters suggest, would have needed training, and 'was probably a keen student of symptoms' – yet the remedies were useless.[8] Why would trained doctors persist in using ineffective remedies, and go to the trouble of writing down their medically useless mixtures for the edification of future doctors? Writing involved considerable expense, both in the creation of the raw materials, and in the time and labour involved in acquiring the examplars and copying them out: commissioning a book was not a task to be undertaken on a whim, and the transmission of texts was, to a significant extent, controlled by the scribes who agreed to write them – scribes who were almost always monks or other ecclesiastic.[9] In this context, it may be worth re-considering the purpose of Anglo-Saxon medicine. Assessments of Anglo-Saxon medicine have traditionally been framed on the assumption that the intention of Anglo-Saxon doctors and their remedies was to cure illness, and on this basis, Anglo-Saxon medical practice has only occasionally been deemed

[1] Grattan and Singer 1952, 94.
[2] Kitson 1989, 65, note 4.
[3] Grendon 1909; Dobbie 1942, 123-4; Storms 1948, 196-203; Scragg 1989; Jolly 1996; Griffiths 1996.
[4] Wright 1955; Cockayne 1864-6.
[5] Grattan and Singer 1952; Payne 1904; Rubin 1974.
[6] Cameron 1983; Cameron 1993; Crawford and Randall 2002.
[7] Brennessel, Drout and Gravel 2005.
[8] *Ibid*, 195.
[9] Brown 2001; Wilcox 2001.

to succeed. Yet the evidence of the documentary sources suggests that, by their own assessment, Anglo-Saxon doctors were confident that their texts were fulfilling the purpose for which they were written. In what follows, archaeological and documentary evidence will be used to try to gain an understanding of Anglo-Saxon perceptions of bodily health and abnormality, and how they responded towards these culturally-negotiated concepts.

Medicine in Anglo-Saxon England from the 5th to the 7th centuries

The period from the arrival of Anglo-Saxon culture in England in the 5th century to the conversion of the Anglo-Saxons to Christianity in the 7th century is essentially prehistoric. No written documents from this period exist to tell us about Anglo-Saxon medicine and health care, but there is a considerable body of archaeological evidence. This gives some indication about intentional activity to control or cure illness or disease, and offers some hints as to what kinds of interventions on the body were practiced at the time, and what kinds of physical differences were the cause of interventions designed to mitigate them.

The chief source of archaeological evidence comes from the many excavated inhumation and cremation cemeteries from this period.[10] Cremation burials from the period, though capable of providing information based on surviving skeletal evidence, are problematic and have been much less intensively studied than the contemporary inhumation burials, which, by contrast, have long been the subject of palaeopathological analysis and discussion.[11] The pre- and proto-Christian Anglo-Saxons practiced furnished inhumation and cremation, where the deceased was interred clothed and sometimes accompanied by artefacts such as vessels, food offerings, weaponry, and jewellery. Variations in the accoutrements associated with the dead allow inferences about the gender, age and status of the dead to be made, even where there is no surviving skeletal evidence.[12]

Individual burials from Anglo-Saxon cemeteries do indicate local and specific examples of attempts to maintain life in the face of difficulties or disincentives in early Anglo-Saxon communities. For example, occasional examples of children and adults with cleft palates, like a 6 year old from Burwell, Cambridgeshire, demonstrate that care was given from birth to babies with physical deviations from the norm. A child born with a cleft palate can breastfeed, but the process is challenging and requires a greater level of effort, and the child from Burwell, for example, was provided with this necessary extra care at birth.[13] Confirmation of a concept of care for sickly infants may have been uncovered in the form of a mammiform pot found during excavation of an inhumation cemetery at Castledyke South, Barton-on-Humber.[14] This artefact, unique in the Anglo-Saxon archaeological record, was found with an infant burial, and may reasonably be interpreted as a feeding bottle.[15] The presence of such an artefact with an infant may suggest that the child was unable to suckle at its mother's breast - either because of a cleft palate, or because its mother could not produce the necessary milk. Because the pot is not paralleled in other Anglo-Saxon graves, its manufacture indicates a specific relationship with the associated infant, and symbolizes that this particular baby was of special importance to its family, both during life and at its early death.

At Worthy Park, Hampshire, grave number 38 offers further evidence of investment of effort into individual health care within Anglo-Saxon communities.[16] This burial was of an adult with a congenital absence of his left arm; it says much for the Anglo-Saxon attitudes towards infants and their survival that this child was helped into adulthood. Similar evidence is suggested by the burial of a possible sufferer of poliomyelitis discovered at the much later 10th century cemetery of Raunds in Northamptonshire.[17] He was a male aged 20-30 years at death, who suffered from the failure of growth of his right femur, right tibia, right fibula, right foot, and tuberculous arthritis of the right knee and left shoulder. His survival of a disease contracted in childhood is indicative of real care of a deformed child. However, these cases only indicate good standards of communal care and welfare for particular individuals. They do not imply specialised medical knowledge.

The majority of diseases and trauma suffered by the early Anglo-Saxons have rarely left any trace in the skeletal record, and any attempts to intervene in the course of these illnesses are equally difficult to see. Even where there is evidence of a wound healing, it is rarely possible to say whether the wound healed with or without some form of intervention. A number of Anglo-Saxon skeletons with head wounds have been identified, for example, and a small proportion of the injuries show signs of healing or having been healed at the time of death, but all might have healed naturally.[18] Evidence for Anglo-Saxon trepanning, however, suggests that the skills existed within the community to treat and successfully heal head wounds. Trepanning was not common in Anglo-Saxon England, but it occurs in a range of contexts from 6th century cemeteries to church cemeteries, with a geographical spread from Kent to Yorkshire, but with a particular cluster of cases around the fenlands, which may have been the work of one practitioner.[19] There is no certainty that trepanning was carried out for 'medical' reasons, in that almost none of the known cases exhibit any sign of pre-existing head wounds or other ailments which might have prompted this

[10] There is no up-to-date database of known early Anglo-Saxon burials, but Audrey Meaney (1964) offers a useful compendium of sites known to that date and indicates the range and richness of early Anglo-Saxon cemeteries. For general overviews of early Anglo-Saxon burial rituals, see for example Lucy 2000, Semple and Williams 2007.

[11] Eg Anglo-Saxon examples of palaeopathology in Brothwell and Higgs 1963, Wells 1964, and detailed studies in eg Wells 1963: for problems in using cremated remains see McKinley 2000.

[12] For discussion of furnished graves and social organisation see Eg. Stoodley 1999, 2000; Dickinson 2002, 2010.

[13] Brothwell 1981 plate 9; see for example Garcez and Guigliano 2005 for a study of breastfeeding success in cleft lip and palate babies: but see the advice of the LaLeche League that a cleft palate baby will not get adequate nutrition through breastfeeding (*Breastfeeding a Baby with a Cleft Lip or Cleft Palate*, La Leche League International, November 2004).

[14] Drinkall and Foreman 1998.

[15] Crawford 1999, 95.

[16] Hawkes and Grainger 2003.

[17] Boddington 1996.

[18] See Boylston 2000, 369-371 for discussion and gazetteer of Anglo-Saxon head injuries.

[19] Parker 1989: Penn 1998.

form of surgery. Typically, the trepanned Anglo-Saxon skulls healed before death, suggesting skill and confidence on the part of the trepanners. The surviving trepanned skulls indicate that it was not for lack of ability that other forms of surgery were not common in the Anglo-Saxon medical repertoire, but that other forms of non-surgical medical treatment were preferred. Recent isolated examples of possible evidence for surgery may alter this perception: a woman from the 9th to 10th century cemetery at Bishopstone, Sussex, excavated in 2004, had cut marks on the bone at the edges of a wound to her knee, indicative of surgery, and Simon Mays has argued for evidence for surgical intervention in the case of another late Anglo-Saxon head wound from Wharram Percy, Yorkshire.[20]

Artefactual evidence for any medical practice beyond basic nurturing of the sick is equally difficult to see in the earlier Anglo-Saxon period. Small metal tool sets known as 'toilet instruments' are found amongst the grave-goods of males and females in this period. They include tiny spoons, tweezers and little picks. It would appear that personal hygiene was of some importance to the Anglo-Saxons, arguably in a ritual context.[21] Perhaps these implements were used to maintain personal appearance, or it may be that there was an awareness that personal hygiene was linked general health. Absent from the Anglo-Saxon archaeological record, however, is anything to compare with the surgical instruments found in Roman contexts.[22] The Anglo-Saxons had some contact with Roman culture, and Germanic troops served in the Roman Army where surgeons practiced their trade, but the Anglo-Saxons do not seem to have inherited or appropriated this aspect of Roman medical practice. In the later documentary evidence too, references to surgical interventions are very few and far between.[23]

What the later documentary sources do show is that herbal treatments - poultices, ointments, creams and drinks - were at the heart of Anglo-Saxon medical theory, and formed the vast majority of recommended treatments. Some of the artefactual evidence from the earlier cemeteries indicates that the herbal tradition dated back to the pre-Christian period. Occasionally, burials are found which include small-lidded canisters, usually with a chain for suspension from a belt, in which fragments of plants or material have been found. These boxes are usually associated with female burials, and it is possible that they represent a small store of healing herbs used by women. It is also possible that these little boxes were amuletic in purpose, and if so, they would form part of a large repertoire of grave goods, including as animal teeth, coins, semi-precious stones, and fossils, which appear to have had a largely amuletic function.[24] Amuletic items of this sort are particularly associated with females, and it may be that in the small dispersed agricultural settlements that dotted the landscape of earlier Anglo-Saxon England, women were the main healers within the community, or they were the ones who depended most heavily on any amuletic or therapeutic function associated with objects such as fossils, stones, teeth and coins.[25]

[20] Schoss, Legge and Thomas 2005; Mays 2005.
[21] Williams 2003.
[22] Jackson 2002, but see also Baker 2004 for a discussion of other uses for Roman medical instruments.
[23] Roberts 1999.
[24] Meaney 1981.

Gender and medicine in the Early Anglo-Saxon period

In the Old English text *Prognostications*, a list of predictions based on a child's date of birth, the fortunes of the male and female child are told. A child born on the fifth moon of the year will, it is predicted, be lucky to survive. After five years; 'he often dies useless. A girl will die worst, because of her evil deeds and witchcraft' (*wyrt-gaelstre* – literally, knowledge of herbs).[26] Other prognostications offer more cheerful prospects: 'the seventeenth moon. None is better for beginning to sow, or for putting children to school. A child born then will be... friendly, sharp, wise, booklearned, bold. A girl will be learned in words (*wordumgelaered*), handy at everything, rich.'[27] Again, 'the twenty-second moon is good for buying servants. A child born on it will be a doctor (*laece*). A girl likewise. And poor.'[28]

It would appear that later, literate Anglo-Saxon society accepted the idea of a witch/wise/medical woman within the community. The semantic variation in the examples cited - '*laece*', '*wordumgelared*', '*wyrt gaelstre*' - might even indicate that there were different, recognized hierarchies or traditions of healing lore, each practice bringing its own rewards.

The archaeological evidence may provide further evidence for women's roles as witches/healers within early Anglo-Saxon society. The first problem posed by the archaeological evidence would rest on how we are to identify the symbols of the medical/magical/religious woman. Bags, pouches, plants and possible amulets do occur in later Anglo-Saxon medical recipes, as do runic or occult letters. In archaeological terms, if the later references to runic writing derive from pre-Christian traditions, the expectation would be to find inscribed items in the grave assemblages of those whose social persona in the mortuary ritual was defined by their special medical skills. In practice, the occurence of runic writing in early Anglo-Saxon contexts is sporadic, and no clear pattern of the distribution of runes, the meanings they were intended to convey, or the purpose of the letters, is identifiable, and the extent to which runic writing was ever considered magical is open to dispute.[29] The difficulty of interpreting the purpose of runic writing is exemplified by one of the earliest English examples, a roe-deer ankle bone found in a fifth century cremation from Caistor-by-Norwich, which has **raihan** (roe-deer) inscribed on the urn: does it help to know that it is what it says it is? As R.I. Page remarked, early Anglo-Saxon runic inscriptions are always 'short, badly preserved and almost always uncertain of meaning'.[30]

While single examples of runic inscriptions on objects may not be helpful, collections of artefacts which may have been thought to have amuletic properties found associated with one body may offer more evidence for a person thought to have

[25] Meaney 1989.
[26] Cockayne 1864-6 Vol 3, 187.
[27] *Ibid*, 193.
[28] *Ibid*, 195.
[29] On the amuletic power of runes, see eg Meaney 1981, 18-23, and Skemer 2006, particularly 44-45, and for an alternative view see eg Page 1964.
[30] Page 1987, 33.

occult or healing power. A woman in the 7th century cemetery at Orsett in Essex, for example, has been identifed as a possible witch, because she had, tied up in a cloth bag, a miscellanaeous collection of oddments whose significance is difficult to explain in terms other than amuletic.[31] The bag contained two copper-alloy pieces from a 7th century hanging bowl, three or more iron rings, an iron guard mount from a knife, a large bead of lignite or shale, and an iron chatelaine.

Was such a collection 'normal' in female graves of this period? An analysis of one rich Kentish cemetery at Buckland, excavated between 1951 and 1965, offers the following results. The excavated area contained about 165 inhumation burials, of which 62 were male and 71 were female. The site was in use between c. 475 until c. 750. Precious materials such as amber, crystal and garnet were found on the site, predominantly with women, because these materials tend to be associated with necklaces which men, within the cemetery ritual, did not possess. 'Amuletic' items in the grave assemblages include fossils, stones not natural to the area, such as iron pyrites, cowrie shells, and various small boxes. 23 burials contained one of the above items, of which only two were male burials - grave C, the burial of a high status male (indicated by the sword included in his grave), whose disturbed grave contained small pebbles, and grave 150, who was buried with a bronze box. It was possible to ascertain the contents of the boxes in only two cases - the remnants of a wooden box apparently enclosed a fossil in the case of grave 55, the burial of a female; and in female burial 60, the box contained a key, two spindle whorls, an amber bead and a large horse tooth. The cemetery site can be divided into chronological plots, according to the dating suggested by the artefacts. Boxes or amulets crop up with women in plots A,B,C,D,E,G,H and I - that is, from the earliest phases of the site to the latest. If one or two women were operating as 'wise women' or 'doctors' within any one generation in a given Anglo-Saxon community, then this is precisely the distribution of items that we would expect. The evidence from the Buckland cemetery would indicate that, while men are not excluded from having amuletic objects, it would appear to be women whose ritual reflects a social status derived from their particular association with the medical or magical amuletic objects.

It is difficult to distinguish between keepsakes and amulets, and it may be that items archaeologists might interpret as 'amuletic' actually had no superstitious significance for their owners, in which case we may say that women, rather than men, were perceived to be the accumulators of such knicknacks in the Buckland burial ritual. There is slender corroborative evidence, however, to indicate that these trinkets may be more than trivial. Burial 67 at Buckland is of a woman whose grave goods include a lump of iron pyrites, but who was buried face down in a contorted position, possibly as a result of having been buried alive.[32] Gruesome though it may appear, this burial is by no means without parallel in the Anglo-Saxon archaeological record. An example comes from the rather poorer Anglian cemetery site at Sewerby, Yorkshire.[33] Grave 41 at this site contained the burials of two women, one on top of the other. The upper was lying face down, her head to the right, her legs and arms raised, with one large stone under her shoulder and part of a beehive quern on her pelvis. She was around 35-45 years of age at the time of her death. Her grave goods include a buckle, knife, jet spindlewhorl, two annular brooches - one bronze, one gilt - some bronze sheet which may have been for suspension, a wooden container, and a string of 15 beads, including amber. She was one of the richest burials in this community, bettered only by one or two burials, including that of the woman buried beneath her - a 17-25 year old, neatly laid out in a wooden coffin. She had sleeve clasps of bronze and gilt (although not a pair) and two strings of beads, one containing 117 beads, including amber and gold, and the other of 88 beads, also including amber and gold.

What is the explanation for this double burial? The prone woman may have been a slave, thrown into the grave after the burial of her owner, but the relatively high-status grave goods associated with her burial undermine this theory. She may have been a sacrifice, although again, her wealth makes this a less attractive theory. Althernatively, she may have been considered responsible in some way for the death of the young woman. The prone woman was buried with a number of items which may have been amuletic: the jet spindle-whorl, the amber beads and the wooden container. These may have been part of the equipment of a witch, and the excavator argued that the most plausible explanation for the events is that the older woman was believed to have caused the death of the younger by misuse of her special knowledge.[34]

Post-conversion medicine in Anglo-Saxon England

Although the majority of the earlier Anglo-Saxons lived a rural, agricultural life, the trading contacts of the elite spread throughout Europe and beyond. By the 7th century, trading contacts with the world beyond England were truly international. The grave goods associated with the early 7th century burial in Mound 1 at Sutton Hoo, Suffolk, included a bronze bowl from Coptic Egypt, silverware from Byzantium, garnet originating from India, and gold coins selected from a range of Frankish mints.[35] From the 7th century onwards, Anglo-Saxon missionaries and royalty were making regular trips to the Continent. Archaeological excavations show widespread 10th century trading contacts. Near Eastern glass has been found in excavations in London, Arabic coins have been found in coin hoards (even a forgery of an Arabic coin in a Viking cess pit at York), pottery containing wine was imported from the Rheinland, quern stones were imported from the Eiffel, and trade (and pilgrims) to the Holy land and Rome were so well established that a part of Rome was known as 'the English quarter'.[36] In terms of art and manuscript production in the later Anglo-Saxon period, English work was arguably the best in Europe, and the colours found in the flowing illustrations of the most expensive examples give some idea of Anglo-Saxon chemical expertise, and offer concrete evidence of access to exotic minerals, including gold, lapis lazuli and

[31] Webster 1985; Meaney 1989, 11.
[32] Evison 1987, 18.
[33] Hirst 1985.
[34] *Ibid*, 40-43.
[35] Bruce-Mitford 1975.
[36] Hall 1984; Vince 1990, 97; Hodges 1989.

silver.[37] To go with the expanding internal and overseas trade, there was a strong monetary system, clear systems of law, taxes and an advanced bureaucracy. The elite of later Anglo-Saxon England were cosmopolitan, urbanised to an extent, and educated.

The catalyst for literacy and the influx of knowledge from the Continent was the Conversion of the Anglo-Saxons to Christianity. The church also became a focus for the healing of diseases, partly as a deliberate process, partly as an inevitable consequence of Christian teaching about the cause of illnesses. The documentary, and, to a lesser extent, archaeological sources for the period, indicate that the church took on a number of roles within the framework of healing. Most spectacular, and most often recorded in the various *Lives* of Anglo-Saxon saints, were the apparently impossible cures and miracles, where the dead were brought to life, prayer cured the sick, and the chronically disabled were healed.

The importance of the church as central to the process of curing disease for the Anglo-Saxons should not be underestimated. According to the teaching of the church, many illnesses were caused by the devil, so a monk, rather than a lay practitioner, was the obvious person to bring health: in a Christian society, ill health and the search for its cure were 'issues of religious, cultural and political significance'.[38] Equally, God himself was considered responsible for punitive illnesses. When thieves attempted to break into the church of the Saint and Martyr St Edmund, for example, the Old English text records that the thieves were struck with paralysis through the night until they were apprehended in the morning and taken away for execution.[39] Again, small wonder that some afflicted with chronic illness hoped that a visit to the church to atone for their sins, or a prayer for the mediation of a powerful saint, might also lead to a cure. One of the most effective saints of the late Anglo-Saxon period was, according to his biographer Aelfric, St Swithun. Prolific miracle cures emanated from his tomb and shrine at the Old Minster, Winchester, which were too numerous in range and quantity for even the keen pen of the hagiographer to record.[40] Amongst Swithun's most noteworthy achievements was the cure of three blind women and their dumb guide; the cure of a paralytic; and the cure of a man who had multiple fractures after a riding accident. According to Aelfric, sick and disabled people would travel considerable distances to seek a cure at Swithun's shrine. One blind English man who had lived for four years in Rome in hope of a miracle from St Peter even travelled back from Rome after being told in a dream that St Swithun would cure him. The power of St Swithun was clearly something of a phenomenon, and crowds gathered at the church for cure. There are indications that Aelfric was not much exaggerating the popularity of this saint, because he described a scene any of his readers could visit for themselves - a church hung about with crutches and cripples' stools from one end to the other, and there were so many of these tokens of Swithun's healing powers that not half of the crutches and stools could be hung up.

[37] Gameson, 1994.
[38] Montserrat 2005, 241.
[39] Skeat 1900, 958-64.
[40] Needham, 1976, 69.

While individual saints gained a reputation for being able to effect miraculous cures, living churchmen were practising medicine and might reasonably be described as doctors. The best recorded of these Anglo-Saxon doctors was St John of Beverley, who died in A.D. 721. His life, written by Bede, is interesting for the way it shows St John distinguishing between cures effected by simple medicine, and miracles. A dumb boy, who was also suffering from a severe skin condition, was brought to the saint to be healed. The hagiographer records that John asked the boy to stick out his tongue. Having made the sign of the cross over the tongue, John asked the boy to repeat after him the sounds of the alphabet, which the boy duly did. Astonished at having found his tongue, the boy, so the hagiographer describes, then spent the rest of the day talking to anyone who would listen. The boy's skin condition, however, is dealt with by 'a physician' (*medico*), who was ordered by Bishop John to undertake the cure of the boy's scabby head.[41] This is medicine. In fact, it is possible that the boy's dumbness was also cured by practical means: if the boy was suffering from the condition known as 'tongue tied', the action of putting his tongue out – particularly if John grasped it to make the sign of the cross – might have broken the frenulum, so effecting a cure.

On another occasion, John's learning is made even more explicit. Visiting an abbess, he was informed that her daughter was fatally ill with a swollen arm, and was asked to make her better. Asking the circumstances of her illness (asking for a history, as any modern family doctor would before attempting a diagnosis), John discovered that the girl had been bled, to which he retorted that: 'You have acted foolishly and ignorantly to bleed her on the fourth day of the moon; I remember how Archbishop Theodore of blessed memory used to say that it was very dangerous to bleed a patient when the moon is waxing and the tide is flowing'.[42]

Archbishop Theodore was sent to England in A.D. 668 by Pope Vitalian. Theodore was a native of Tarsus in Cilicia, and was 'well trained in secular and divine literature, both Greek and Latin'.[43] It was through such men that Greek and Latin literature, including medical literature, was brought to the Anglo-Saxons, and Bishop John was a product of their training.[44] John's miracles, as recorded by Bede, illustrate that the Greek and Roman medical tradition was alive and working in 7th century Anglo-Saxon England, and that it was a first course of action in the case of illness. Only when it was clear that 'conventional' medicine would fail, would miracles be resorted to.

Behind this show of miracles, there is evidence that some churchmen had more formal training in medicine, and were knowledgeable doctors within the Roman tradition, with some access to the standard classical medical texts. In addition, cemetery evidence suggests that the church took on the long-term care of the chronically sick. There is some further archaeological evidence to suggest that the church functioned as the primary carer for the sick in some circumstances.

[41] Colgrave and Mynors 1969, 457-459.
[42] *Ibid*, 461.
[43] *Ibid*, 331.
[44] Wilson 2006, 23.

One cemetery associated with a nunnery at Nazeingby, Northamptonshire, included the burial of a severely disabled older adult, suffering from possible congenital dislocation of the hips. According to the site report, 'there is no way in which this man could have reached the age of 50 without a great deal of help'.[45] Further skeletons with relatively high levels of bone pathology were also found in this cemetery, including a female aged over 50 years with very bad osteo-arthritis; a female over 50 with osteo-arthritis and bone changes typical of tuberculosis; a male burial aged between 35 and 45 with fatigue fractures of both feet; a case of hydrocephalus aged between 25 and 30 at the time of death; and a case of Down's syndrome.[46] The population within this cemetery was highly unusual, and the preponderance of females, together with the extreme old age of many of the burials, and the degree of caring for the sick demonstrated by the survival into old age of some of the highly pathological individuals, suggests that this is the cemetery of a hospice run by a religious order.[47]

Secular medicine in Later Anglo-Saxon England

On the continent, there is evidence that Merovingian Frankish kings, bishops and nobility had ready access to lay, trained medical attendants.[48] There was a great deal of contact between the Kings of Anglo-Saxon England and Francia (the mission of St Augustine to England in 597 gained an easy entry into Kent because the Kentish king Ethelbert was married to the Frankish princess Bertha), but there is little evidence for such courtly doctors in Anglo-Saxon documents.

The problem of identifying medicine in a non-ecclesiastical setting in Anglo-Saxon England is compounded by the fact that all known scriptoria were ecclesiastical, so it would seem likely that the surviving Old English medical texts were produced in a monastic setting.[49] However, the people mentioned by name who appear to have special medical knowledge may well have been secular. The four most likely contenders for the role of 'doctor' in late Anglo-Saxon England are all found in the Old English medical text known as Bald's *Leechbook*. The style of Bald's *Leechbook* indicates that it was intended as an *aide memoire* for someone familiar with the subject matter.[50] A great deal of knowledge on the part of the reader is assumed, to such an extent that it seems very likely that the book represents the personal text of a medical practitioner, probably Bald himself. The skill of the copyist, Cild, suggests that he, too, may have had some medical knowledge or training.[51]

Bald's *Leechbook* is not an 'original' work, any more than a modern medical textbook is, and its acknowledgement within the text of the work of other doctors provides us with two more personal names, 'Oxa' and 'Dun', both males. 'Other doctors' are not always Anglo-Saxons, however. Parts of the *Leechbook* are derived from the *Medicina Plinii, Practica Alexandri* and other texts. In Book II, the contents list says that information on the liver is provided by 'doctors [who] teach this remedy for swelling and injury to the liver', and 'doctors say these are the symptoms of a swollen and damaged liver, and remedies for that, and for hardening of the liver'. Malcolm Cameron has shown that these remedies are a close translation of the *Epitome Altera* of Vindicianus.[52] Sometimes, the sources are acknowledged within the text. In *Leechbook* Book I, 87:1, the 'Great Doctor Plinius' is referenced.[53] However, Bald does not particularly discriminate between the medical knowledge and authority of his native and continental sources.

Bald may not have had had direct access to the Mediterranean works he translates, and he may have been drawing on other Old English translations of translations.[54] However he came by his information, Bald was pulling together the known and tried knowledge of all doctors, pooling sources to provide an up-to-date compendium of 10th century medical practice. It is impossible to tell to what extent Bald dictated the collection of material found in the text, nor whether the scribe Cild understood the source material he was copying, although comparing some of the original sources to the Anglo-Saxon versions, it would seem that both had some knowledge of what they were about - foreign ingredients have been swapped for herbs available in England, and editing and selection of the original sources has taken place.[55]

***Bald's* Leechbook**

Bald's *Leechbook* provides an invaluable insight into the medical knowledge-base of the day, showing that, while there was a strong influence from the Graeco-Roman system of medicine, the Anglo-Saxon practitioner was not an ignorant or uncritical follower of foreign texts. Bald's carefully-organised collection of remedies drew on experience and other, native medical traditions, too. The scriptorium at Winchester may well have been responsible for producing Bald's *Leechbook*. The surviving copy of the *Leechbook* (there may once have been many) is in the British Museum, MS Royal 12 D.xvii, and is available in facsimile.[56] The surviving manuscript of Bald's *Leechbook* consists of three sections or books, the first two of which are thought to belong together, and seem to form an intentional whole. The third book may have been a later addition.[57]

Book I follows standard Graeco-Roman practice in being divided up into a logical sequence, starting with illnesses of the head and moving progressively around the body. Sections 1 - 13 of Book I cover diseases of the head, including eye problems, coughs, deafness and nosebleeds. Sections 14 - 22 discuss diseases of the body, from coughs and vomiting to unspecific pains in the sides up to 'pain in the loins'. This leads on to leg problems, which are dealt with in sections 23 to 30, again ranging from the relatively minor (chilblains and over-exercising), to severe (splinting a broken leg). Sections 31 to 44 give information on how to treat diseases that affect the whole body, such as jaundice, cancer and gangrene. The odd

[45] Huggins 1978, 57.
[46] *Ibid*, 57.
[47] *Ibid*, 63.
[48] Thorpe 1974, 191, 263, 269, 407, 463.
[49] Wilcox 2001.
[50] Brennessel, Drout and Gravel 2005.
[51] Cameron 1993, 21, 33.

[52] *Ibid*, 93.
[53] Cockayne 1864-6 Vol 1, 155.
[54] Cameron 1993, 83-92.
[55] *Ibid*.
[56] Wright 1955.
[57] *Ibid*.

exception is section 34, where remedies for apparently trivial nail problems nestle in between remedies for ulcerating skin and remedies for 'blackened and deadened body'. Sections 45 to 54 are about 'worm' diseases; that is, illnesses that either were, or were believed to have been, caused by insects or parasites. Remedies 55 to 61 are concerned with paralysis of one sort or another, while remedies 62 to 67 are about fevers and madness. The remaining remedies are an eclectic group, made up of the 'leftovers' - diseases or problems that do not obviously fit into any of the other categories, such as dog bite, impotence and bloodletting (the most common surgical procedure of the day). Book II is concerned with internal ailments.

Although the books seem to be given a logical order, the actual remedies for any given problem seem to be offered in a heap, with no way of differentiating between them. In the first section of Book I, for example, there are twelve remedies for 'a headache', each offering a different range of herbal treatments, including drinks, pastes and creams derived from both native and exotic plants:

> Rub a penny weight of the plant called myrrh in a mortar, add a bucket full of wine to the pulp, rub the head with it and drink it at night fasting. For headache, take rue and wormwood, pound and mix with vinegar and oil, sieve through a cloth, rub it onto the head, or make a paste with the same ingredients, apply it to the head, and cover it with bandages when you want to go to bed. For the same thing, take betony and pepper, rub thoroughly together, leave them hanging up in a cloth overnight, use as a cream.[58]

There is no hint that one of these - and the list goes on for another nine remedies 'for the same thing' - is any more efficacious than another, nor any hint of differentiation between these headaches, yet headaches are caused by a variety of illnesses, and lead to a variety of associated symptoms.[59] Headaches may be throbbing, persistent, sharp, or associated with dizziness and nausea. Headaches may be caused by anything from a trivial hangover to a life threatening brain tumour. The Anglo-Saxon doctor, if using Bald's *Leechbook* as his only source, can deal only with the one symptom, and apparently cannot identify different remedies for the different causes. This may offer an explanation for the wide range of remedies for what are seemingly the same diseases. For headache, which could have a variety of causes, a range of remedies was appropriate, because one or the other of them might eventually be efficacious. Read in this way, the *Leechbook*, if it is supposed to offering advice, seems to be advocating a muddled 'lottery methodology' in medicine - keep trying, because one day you might hit the right combination.

However, what a reading of the whole manuscript shows is that there may have been a conscious choice not to include the details we might expect, because occasionally they are included: remedies for nausea (19) and, swelling (41) are described as 'noble'; those for spider bite (68) are 'excellent', and that for 'blackened and deadened body' (gangrene) are described as 'powerful and noble remedies' (35). It may well be, then, that the Old English medical text appears muddled because it was written for a trained doctor who would know how to differentiate between the remedies in a way lost to the modern, ignorant reader.

It is also clear from the descriptions within the *Leechbook* that the Anglo-Saxon doctor was perfectly capable of observing symptoms and the progress of some diseases. The accurate descriptions of gangrene and jaundice are testimony to this skill, as is the following useful and reasonable treatment for a fractured skull:

> For a fractured skull, and if the brain is visible, mix a little egg yolk with honey, fill the wound with it, cover with a bandage of hemp. Then leave it alone, and after about three days look at the wound. If there is a red ring in the healthy skin around the wound, then you will know that it is incurable.[60]

Furthermore, there are some remedies where distinctions between types of ailment are made by simple tests. For a swollen throat, windpipe and mouth, the reader is advised that:

> There are two types of the disease. One is in the jaws: when you look into the open mouth it is swollen and is red about the uvula, and the patient cannot breathe easily and feels suffocated, also he cannot swallow or speak easily, and has lost his voice. However the disease is not dangerous. The other is when the throat is swollen and pussy, the patient cannot speak, and the swelling is in both the neck and the tongue. The patient is unable to breathe easily and cannot turn his neck, or lean his head forward to see his navel, and unless he is treated immediately he will be dead in about three days.[61]

Here, there is advice on how to predict the progress of the disease, and how to distinguish between serious and less serious illnesses when the patient presents similar symptoms. A final example of this, and perhaps the most impressive, is the section on the treatment of gangrene:

> If the swelling skin eruptions or the red mould come externally from wounds or cuts or blows, treat the condition immediately with scarification and applications of barley, in the way that knowledgeable doctors well know how; you will make it better. If the blackened area is so deadened that there is no feeling in it, then you must immediately cut away all the dead and numb parts to the living body so that none of the dead area is left of that which could feel neither ice (iron?) nor fire before. After that, treat the wound as you would the part that still has some sensation and is not completely dead. You must draw the blood from the deadened place with frequent scarifyings, sometimes severe, sometimes light. If you must chop or cut an unsound limb from a healthy body, then do not cut on the border of the healthy area, but cut into the well and healthy area so that you will make it better and cure it more quickly. Treat the cuts like this: take bean meal or oat meal or barley meal,

[58] Cockayne 1864-6 Vol 1, 19.

[59] The compiler does distinguish between 'headache' from 'half a headache', for which there is a similarly long list of remedies.

[60] Cockayne 1864-6 Vol 1, 83, 107, 23, translations by the author.

[61] *Ibid*, 47.

> or such meal as you think will do to apply, add vinegar and honey, cook together and apply and bandage on to the sore places. If you want the ointment to be more powerful, add a little salt to it and bandage it up now and then, and bathe with vinegar or with wine. If needs be, give a herbal drink occasionally.[62]

Such careful and accurate instructions, asking the doctor to use discretion and observation, are well within the Mediterranean tradition of 'rational' medicine. Aspects of Anglo-Saxon medical knowledge mirrored the best available anywhere in the pre-modern world at the time. If other remedies do not describe illnesses in detail, or differentiate remedies for the same illness, it would seem that it was not because the compiler of the *Leechbook* was incapable of such thought processes, but that he chose not to in most cases. In this context, why did well-educated Anglo-Saxon medical practitioners choose to incorporate the kind of 'superstitious' material into their lexicon, which has given Anglo-Saxon medicine such a poor reputation?

Magic and Anglo-Saxon medical theory

Bald was neither a charlatan nor a superstitious simpleton, and the bulk of his remedies offer practical, or at least non-occult, medical provision. It is noticeable that charms and chants make up only a tiny proportion of the remedies. Magic and chanting are given the least important place in the manuscript. Recipes that rely heavily on chants and ritualised magic within Bald's *Leechbook* are almost always for ailments where there was little that herbs or medicinal knowledge could do to help the process. In other Old English medical texts, the same observation applies. One remedy in the *Herbarium Apuleii* for easy childbirth is of a quasi-medical type:

> In order that a woman may give birth quickly, take seed of this same coriander, eleven grains or thirteen, knit them, with a thread on a clean linen cloth let then a person who is a virgin, a boy or a girl, take them and hold this at the left thigh, and as soon as the birth is over, take away the medicine in case part of the insides follow after.[63]

There is no likelihood of this remedy having any medical effect whatsoever; although it may be that the detailed instructions and the warning about the efficacy of the treatment had a powerful psychological value. Other remedies reveal all too clearly the underlying helplessness of the medical practitioner. In just the same way that the most intractable modern diseases spawn the widest range of solutions - there are over 80 preparations on the market for arthritic complaints - in the same way the least treatable early medieval ailments seem to have generated the most complicated, extravagant or occult remedies - cancers, fevers and childbirth fall into this category. In the *Lacnunga*, a less 'rational' collection of remedies than Bald's *Leechbook*, a woman who cannot give birth to her child is to step over the grave of a dead man three times offering a chant, then over her sleeping husband, and then is to go to church. Ultimately, if she cannot give birth to live children, she is to: 'take a bit of her own child's grave and wrap it in black wool and sell it to the trader and then say; I sell it, I have sold it, this black wool and these grains of sorrow'.[64] Similarly, a woman who cannot give birth is to spit milk over running water, and to enter another dwelling to the one she left.[65] Both remedies are in the tradition of folk medicine on the basis of charms and amulets, and are not borrowed from a classical model, but both, typically, deal with a medical problem that was beyond the reach of any tradition of medical knowledge at the time. A complicated charm at least had the virtue of doing the woman little harm, while offering some palliative comfort.[66]

Conclusions

To say that 'magic' formed part of 'rational' Anglo-Saxon medicine only as a last resort, tempting though it is in terms of reclaiming the Anglo-Saxons from the 'Dark Ages' of medical history, does not provide a complete picture of the true ethos behind the inclusive Anglo-Saxon attitudes towards medicine. First, it seems that ownership of healing knowledge was differently gendered at different times in the Anglo-Saxon period. The availability of knowledge and care was also fluid: where access to any medicine was limited, pragmatic – or, in the case of the Castledyke feeding bottle, sympathetic - care co-existed with other genres of treatment. Christianity brought with it new negotiations about the role of men and women in relationship to knowledge of health and healing. The later texts also indicate that medicinal knowledge had a place within a more complex framework which had more to do with a philosophy of knowledge than with medicine.

As Bald's *Leechbook* makes clear, those who had access to medical knowledge in Anglo-Saxon England were expected to behave, in many ways, like their modern counterparts. Case histories might be taken, and the doctor was supposed to use discretion and observation in the prescribing of dosages: for gangrene the medical practitioner is counselled to take stock, and to think about the patient rather than mechanically prescribing according to the book:

> ...always consider when you are giving potent medicines what the strength and condition of the patient is. Are they strong or vigorous, so that they can cope with strong medicine, or are they delicate and frail and weak, so that they will not be able to stand the medicine. Apply the medicine according to the condition of the patient, because there is a great difference between the bodies of men, women and children, and in the strength of the daily labourer and the leisured, of the old and the young and of those used to hardships and those who are unused to such circumstances. It is a fact that a pale body is weaker and tenderer than tanned and sunburnt ones. If you intend to cut a limb from the body, then consider the condition of the area and the strength of the place, because some areas fester more readily if they are not carefully attended. Some react to the treatment later, some sooner.[67]

---

[62] *Ibid*, 83.
[63] Cockayne 1864-6 Vol 2, 219.
[64] Cockayne, 1864-6 Vol 3, 67.
[65] *Ibid*, 69.
[66] Rubin 1974.
[67] Cockayne 1864-6 Vol 1, 83.

This medical advice appears startlingly 'modern' and 'rational', and on one level, it is. However, this very same advice is echoed in a 10th century law code of King Aethelred, who was strongly influenced by Archbishop Wulfstan of York:

> And always the greater a man's position in this present life, or the higher the privileges of his rank, the more fully shall he make amends for his sins, and the more dearly shall he pay for all misdeeds; for the strong and the weak are not alike, nor can they bear a like burden, any more than the sick can be treated like the sound. And therefore, in forming a judgment, careful discrimination must be made between age and youth, wealth and poverty, health and sickness, and the various ranks of life.[68]

The similarities between the medical text on the one hand, and the law code on the other, are a timely reminder that physical health, mental health, spiritual health, and the health of the kingdom, were not separate entities, to be partitioned in the Anglo-Saxon mind. The elite of Anglo-Saxon society, trained in Latin and Greek by the church and through church schools, but writing confidently and fluently in their own language too (a rarity in Early Medieval Europe), viewed medical knowledge, the ability to heal the physical body, not as a skill separate from political skill or religious knowledge, but as an intrinsic part of the wider pool of all human knowledge, knowledge which, in turn, when written down, became part of a wider Christian exercise in collating information, whether historical, geographical, or medicinal, which could help to explain God's ways to man. In this way, Bede's *Ecclesiastical History of the English People* is useful history, but its primary intention is to demonstrate the work of God, and it draws on both documentary sources and oral tradition to do so. Similarly, an Old English collection of texts on monsters such as *Wonders of the East* drew on an eclectic mix of learned Latin writing, popular tradition, and native folklore.[69] Anglo-Saxon medical texts, like other genres of writing for the period, were vehicles for the 'revelation of the unknowable God, or... for the revalation of the fundamentally real'.[70] It is in this context that Anglo-Saxon medical texts should be judged.

Bibliography

Baker, P. 2004. 'Roman Medical Instruments: Archaeological Interpretations of their Possible "Non-functional uses"', *Journal of the Social History of Medicine*,**17**, 3-21.

Boddington, A. 1996. *Raunds Furnells: the Anglo-Saxon Church and Churchyard: Raunds Area Project,* English Heritage Archaeological Report 7, London: English Heritage.

Brennessel, B., Drout, M. and Gravel, R. 2005. 'A reassessment of the efficacy of Anglo-Saxon medicine,' *Anglo-Saxon England*, **34**, 183-195.

Brothwell, D. 1981. *Digging up Bones: the excavation, treatment and study of human skeletal remains*, Oxford: Oxford University Press.

Brothwell, D. and Higgs, E. 1963. *Science in archaeology*, London: Thames and Hudson.

Brown, M.P. 2001. 'Anglo-Saxon manuscript production: issues of making and using', in P. Pulsiano and E. Treharne (eds), *A companion to Anglo-Saxon literature*, Oxford: Blackwell.

Bruce-Mitford, R. 1975. *The Sutton Hoo Ship-Burial: Volume 1. Excavations, Background, the ship, dating and inventory*, London: British Museum Publications Limited.

Boylston, A. 2000. Evidence for weapon-related trauma in British archaeological samples', in M. Cox and S. Mays (eds), *Human osteology in archaeology and forensic science*, 357-380, Cambridge: Cambridge University Press.

Cameron, M.L. 1983. 'The sources of medical knowledge in Anglo-Saxon England', *Anglo-Saxon England*, **11**,135-55.

Cameron, M. 1993. *Anglo-Saxon Medicine*, Cambridge: Cambridge University Press.

Cockayne, O. 1864-6. *Leechdoms, Wortcunning and Starcraft of Early England*, 3 volumes, London.

Crawford, S. 1999. *Childhood in Anglo-Saxon England*, Stroud: Sutton.

Crawford, S. and Randall, A. 2002. 'Bald's *Leechbook* and archaeology: two approaches to Anglo-Saxon health and healthcare' in R. Arnott (ed.), *The Archaeology of Medicine: Papers given at a session of the annual conference of the Theoretical Archaeology Group held at the University of Birmingham on 20 December 1998*, British Archaeology Report International Series 1046, 101-104, Oxford: BAR Publishing.

Colgrave, B. and Mynors, R. 1969. *Bede: Ecclesiastical History of the English People*, Oxford: Oxford University Press.

Dickinson, T, 2002. 'Review article: What's New in Early Medieval Burial Archaeology?', *Early Medieval Europe*, **11(1)**, 71–87.

Dickinson, T. 2010. 'Mortuary ritual: overview', in H. Hamerow, D. Hinton and S. Crawford, (eds.), *The Oxford Handbook of Anglo-Saxon Archaeology*, 223-39, Oxford: Oxford University Press.

Dobbie, E.V.K. 1942. *The Anglo-Saxon Minor Poems*, Anglo-Saxon Poetic Records 6, New York: Columbia University Press.

Drinkall, G. and Foreman, M. 1998. *The Anglo-Saxon cemetery at Castledyke South, Barton-on-Humber*, Sheffield: Sheffield Academic Press.

Evison, V.I. 1987. *Dover: Buckland Anglo-Saxon Cemetery*, Historic Buildings and Monuments Commission for England Archaeological Report no 3.

Gameson, R. (ed.) 1994. *The Early Medieval Bible: its production, decoration and use*, Cambridge studies in Palaeography and codicology 2, Cambridge: Cambridge University Press.

Garcez L.W. and Giugliani E.R. 2005. 'Population-based study on the practice of breastfeeding in children born with cleft lip and palate', *Cleft Palate Craniofacial Journal,* **42(6)**, 687-93.

Grattan, J.H.G. and Singer, C. 1952. *Anglo-Saxon Magic and Medicine: illustrated specially from the semi-pagan text 'Lacnunga'*, Publications of the Wellcome Historical Medical Museum 3, London: Geoffrey Cumberlege.

[68] Robertson 1925, 9.
[69] Orchard 1995, 22.
[70] Williams 1996, 286.

Grendon, F. 1909. 'The Anglo-Saxon Charms', *Journal of American Folk-Lore*, **22**, 105-237.

Griffiths, B. 1996. *Aspects of Anglo-Saxon Magic*, Norfolk: Anglo-Saxon Books.

Hall, R.A. 1984. *The Viking Dig: the excavations at York*, London: Bodley Head.

Hawkes, S.C. and Grainger, G. 2003. *The Anglo-Saxon cemetery at Worthy Park, Kingsworthy, near Winchester, Hampshire*, Oxford University School of Archaeology Monograph 59.

Hirst, S. 1985. *An Anglo-Saxon Inhumation Cemetery at Sewerby, East Yorkshire*, York University Archaeological Publications 4.

Hodges, R. 1989. *Dark Age Economics: The origins of towns and trade, A.D. 600-1000*, 2nd edit., London: Duckworth,

Huggins, P.J. 1978. 'Excavations of a Belgic and Romano-British farm with Middle Saxon cemetery and churches at Nazeingbury, Essex, 1975-6', *Essex Archaeology and History*, 3rd Series, **32**, 63-96.

Jackson, R. 2002. 'Roman surgery: the evidence of the instruments', in R. Arnott (ed.), *The archaeology of medicine: papers given at a session of the annual conference of the theoretical Archaeology Group held at the University of Birmingham on 20 December 1998*, 87-94, British Archaeological Reports International Series 1046, Oxford: BAR Publishing.

Jolly, K.L. 1996. *Popular religion in late Anglo-Saxon England: elf charms in context*, Chapel Hill: University of North Carolina Press.

Kitson, P. 1989. 'From eastern learning to Western folklore; the transmission of some medico-magical ideas' in D. Scragg (ed.), *Superstition and popular magic in Anglo-Saxon England*, 57-71, Manchester: Manchester University Press.

Lucy, S. 2000. *The Anglo-Saxon Way of Death*. Stroud: Sutton.

McKinley, J. 2000. 'The analysis of cremated bone' in M. Cox and S. Mays (eds), *Human osteology in archaeology and forensic science*, 403-422, Cambridge: Cambridge University Press.

Mays, S. 'A possible case of surgical treatment of cranial blunt force injury from medieval England' *International Journal of Osteoarchaeology*, **16:2**, 95-103.

Meaney, A.L. 1964. *A Gazetteer of early Anglo-Saxon burial sites*, London: Allen and Unwin.

Meaney, A.L. 1981, *Anglo-Saxon Amulets and Curing Stones*, British Archaeological Reports British Series 96, Oxford: British Archaeological Reports.

Meaney, A.L. 1989. 'Women, witchcraft and magic in Anglo-Saxon England', in D. Scragg, (ed.), *Superstition and popular magic in Anglo-Saxon England*, 9-40, Manchester: Manchester University Press.

Montserrat, D. 2005. 'Carrying on the work of the earlier firm: doctors, medicine and Christianity in the *Thaumata* of Sophronius of Jerusalem', in H. King (ed.), *Health in Antiquity*, 230-242, London: Routledge.

Needham, G.I. (ed.) 1976. *Aelfric: Lives of Three English Saints*, Exeter: Exeter University Press.

Orchard, A. 1995. *Pride and prodigies: studies in the monsters of the Beowulf manuscript*, London: D.S. Brewer.

Page, R.I. 1964. 'Anglo-Saxon runes and magic', *Journal of the British Archaeological Association*, 3rd series, **27**, 14-31.

Page, R.I., 1987. *Reading' the Past: Runes*, London: British Museum Press.

Parker, S.J. 1989. 'Skulls, symbols and surgery: a review of the evidence for trepanation in Anglo-Saxon England and a consideration of the motives behind the practice' in D. Scragg, (ed.), *Superstition and popular magic in Anglo-Saxon England*, 73-84, Manchester: Manchester University Press.

Payne, S. 1904. *English Medicine in Anglo-Saxon Times: two lectures delivered before the Royal college of physicians of London, June 23 and 25, 1903*, Oxford: Clarendon Press.

Penn, K. 1998. *An Anglo-Saxon cemetery at Oxborough, West Norfolk, excavations in 1990*, East Anglian Archaeology Occasional Papers no 5, Bury St Edmunds: East Anglian Archaeology.

Roberts, C. 1999. 'Surgery', in Lapidge, M., Blair, J., Keynes, S., and Scragg, D. (eds), *The Blackwell Encyclopedia of Anglo-Saxon England*, 430-431, Oxford: Blackwells.

Robertson, A.J. (ed. and trans.) 1925. *The Laws of the Kings of England from Edmund to Henry I: Part I: Edmund to Canute*, Cambridge: Cambridge University Press.

Rubin, S. 1974. *Medieval English Medicine*, Newton Abbot: David and Charles.

Schoss, L. C. D., Legge, S.S., and Thomas, G. 2005. 'A case of Anglo-Saxon knee surgery?', paper delivered at the 7th Annual Conference of the British Association for Biological Anthropology and Osteoarchaeology. London, U.K.. Jan. 2005.

Scragg, D.G. (ed.) 1989. *Superstition and popular magic in Anglo-Saxon England*, Manchester: Manchester University Press.

Semple, S. and Williams, H. (eds) 2007. *Early Medieval Mortuary Practices*. Anglo-Saxon Studies in Archaeology and History 14. Oxford: Oxford University Committee for Archaeology.

Skeat, W.W. (ed.) 1900. *Aelfric's Lives of the Saints* ii, Early English Text Society Original Series 114, London.

Skemer, D.C. 2006 *Binding words: textual amulets in the Middle Ages*, Pennsylvania: Pennsylvania State University Press.

Stoodley, N. 1999 *The Spindle and the Spear: a Critical Enquiry into the Construction and Meaning of Gender in the early Anglo-Saxon Burial Rite*, BAR British Series, Oxford: BAR Publishing.

Stoodley, N. 2000. 'From the cradle to the grave: age organisation and the early Anglo-Saxon burial rite', *World Archaeology*, **31.3**, 456-472.

Storms, G. 1948. *Anglo-Saxon Magic,* The Hague: Martinus Nijhoff.

Thorpe, L. (trans.) 1974. *Gregory of Tours; The History of the Franks*. London: Penguin.

Vince, A. 1990. *Saxon London: An Archaeological investigation*, London: Seaby.

Webster, L. 1985. 'The grave goods', in J.D. Hedges and D.G. Buckley, 'Anglo-Saxon burials and later features excavated at Orsett, Essex, 1975', *Medieval Archaeology*, **29**, 8-13.

Wells, C. 1963. 'Polyostotic Fibrous Dysplasia in a Seventh-century Anglo-Saxon', *British Journal of Radiology*, **36**, 925-926.

Wells, C. 1964. *Bones, bodies and disease*. London: Thames and Hudson.

Wilcox, J. 2001. 'Transmission of literature and learning: Anglo-Saxon scribal culture', in P. Pulsiano and E. Treharne (eds), *A companion to Anglo-Saxon literature*, Oxford: Blackwell.

Williams, D. 1996. *Deformed discourse: the function of the monster in mediaeval thought and literature*, Montreal: McGill-Queen's University Press.

Williams, H. 2003. 'Material culture as memory: combs and cremation in early Medieval Britain,' *Early Medieval Europe*, **12(2)**, 89-128.

Wilson, S.E. 2006. *The life and after-life of St John of Beverley: the evolution of a cult of an Anglo-Saxon saint*, Aldershot: Ashgate publishing.

Wright, C.E. 1955. *Bald's Leechbook*, Early English Manuscript Facsimiles 5, Copenhagen: Rosenkilde and Bagger.

Chapter Six

'This should not to be shown to a gentile': Medico-Magical Texts in Medieval Franco-German Jewish Rabbinic Manuscripts

Ephraim Shoham-Steiner

Introduction

In a recently published volume of collected essays titled: 'The Jews of Europe in the Middle Ages', Anna Sapir-Abulafia wrote the following:

> Until recently much of this work [referring to the historiographical attempts to map the major developments that took place in Europe between 1000-1300] has concentrated almost exclusively on the majority society of Latin Christendom i.e. Catholics. As interest has grown in the neglected groups among those Catholics, as for example woman and the illiterate, Historians have widened their horizons to look beyond the narrow confines of institutional Catholicism in order to investigate so called "outsiders" like heretics Jews and Muslims...The more we find out about Medieval Jewry, the more we are struck by the extent to which Jews were a significant players in all facets of life of their host societies.[1]

In this article, as in my entire research agenda, I follow a similar lead and wish to speak not only of Jews but about their relationship and exchange with their respective Christian neighbours. Previous scholarship has pointed out a trope that received the catchy name *La Convivencia*, namely the mutual co-existence of Christians, Muslims and Jews during the Middle Ages in the Iberian Peninsula, and the relatively good relationship between individuals from all three denominations. Historiography has adopted this trope and identified the Iberian realm as the site where one should expect cultural exchange to take, by contrast to the rest of western Europe.[2] I therefore set my gaze and scholarly interest on the geographic areas 'less expected' for cultural exchange, namely England, Northern France, and the *Regum Teutonicum*. My previous research focused on marginal individuals in medieval Franco-German (henceforth: Ashkenazi) Jewish society.[3] In this article I would like to look at another 'marginal' phenomenon: the marginal notations found in many medieval Franco-German Hebrew manuscripts. Examination of these notations, or insertions made 'in the blanks', reveals an abundance of re-copied charms, and a variety of additional medical, magical, or practical advice.

A few remarks are required. First, it should be noted that the world of medieval Jewish manuscripts, as rich and variegated as it may be, falls dramatically short in quantity compared to its contemporary Christian counterpart. Jewish communities were a minority society within the western European framework, and although the percentage of literate individuals within the communities was probably higher then that of their Christian neighbours, nevertheless the actual numbers are dramatically smaller. Moreover we should bear in mind that most of the material found in the main body of the text of these manuscripts represents the cultural concerns of the learned Jewish rabbinic elite penned in Hebrew, the learned elite's *lingua franca*. Thus a great portion of the medico-magical material which will be the focus of our discussion was penned on the margins of texts with a religious orientation: Talmudic texts, biblical hermeneutical and homiletic texts, religious and legal *responsa* literature, and liturgical texts as well. Nevertheless we shouldn't assume (incorrectly) that the phenomenon under discussion is a negligible or marginal one – on the contrary. Such notations are a common phenomenon and appear in many medieval Franco-German manuscripts. The purpose of this paper is to shed some light on this material and provide it with the scholarly attention it deserves.

In order to illustrate the phenomenon in question, an example is needed. In the blank space between the end of an anonymous commentary on the Pentateuch and the next rabbinic text from MS Parma, Bibliotheca Palatina Heb. 2342, we find a single notation: a remedy to cure a troubling earache. Although the handwritings differ, palaeographical considerations indicate that the remedy was written not long after the main body of the text in the same calligraphy style common among Ashkenazi Jews in the 13th and 14th centuries. The remedy reads as follows: 'To clear the ear: take the milk of a nursing she-dog and drip it into the ear and it will heal, with God's help.' MS Parma 2342, or as it was previously known, De Rossi 541, is a large 13th century Ashkenazi manuscript in which almost every genre of Ashkenazi writing is represented. Apparently half of a larger codex that was split in the late Middle Ages or in early Modern times, probably for commercial reasons, its 16th century colophon reveals that it belonged to a Venetian Jew of Ashkenazi descent by the name of Kalonymus ben

[1] Abulafia 2004, 19. On the role of medieval Jewry in medieval history, see Skinner 2003, 219-247.

[2] For a fine articulation of the historiographical opinions regarding intercultural exchange verses insularity tendencies among medieval Jews and their surroundings and the real or imagined difference between the medieval Franco-German realm (*Ashkenaz*) and the Iberian peninsula (*Sepharad*), see Malkiel 2007.

[3] Shoham-Steiner 2007.

Mordechai Cohen.[4]

The texts compiled in MS Parma 2342 represent typical medieval Ashkenazi rabbinic material. To name a few of the works found in this manuscript : (1) the aforementioned rather lengthy, 107-page-long anonymous commentary on the Pentateuch, (2) an Ashkenazi legal work on the laws of menstrual ritual impurity (Niddah), (3) a fragmentary commentary on the prayer book (the scribe decided to copy only the parts he found relevant to his needs); (4) a small collection of late antiquity Jewish homiletic texts known as Midrashim Ketanim; (5) eclectic legal responses of various Jewish Ashkenazi legal authorities, and so on. Parma 2342 is also rather typical from the paleographical perspective. Written in several hands, it was either compiled piecemeal, or bound together by a later editor who wished to compile its different works together in a single codex. Nonetheless, all its different hands exhibit the paleographical characteristic features of 13th- to 14th-century Ashkenazi handwriting.

It should be noted at this early point in our discussion that this marginal 'medical' material differs greatly from the medical know-how found in 'conventional' medieval Hebrew medical tractates. By 'conventional' medical tractates I refer to works like: The Book of Asaf the Physician; Hebrew translations of Avicenna's Canon; the 14th century Provençal Hebrew translations of the work of Bernard de Gordon of Montpellier (*Lilium Medicine*); or Maimonides's Shem-Tov ben Joseph ibn Falaquera (also spelled Palquera) and Isaac Israeli's medical writings. As opposed to these systematic medical treatises, which follow Arabic Greek-Byzantine and medieval European medical traditions, the marginal entries that are the concern of this paper contain no long lists of ailments, no elaborate anatomical descriptions, and no detailed lists of *materia medica*.[5]

Here we shall concern ourselves with other kinds of medical know-how that are far less systematic and philosophical but of no less social importance. First I will describe this 'marginal' material and convey something of the flavour of these texts. Then I wish to address certain problems that arise, especially the ostensible contradiction between the nature of some of these texts and the main textual components of the manuscripts in which they appear. Finally, I will argue that the wide range of texts penned in the blanks and in the margins of manuscripts were either in actual everyday use, or, at the very least, thought worthy of being recorded and made available for everyday use. I submit that analysis of these materials, largely overlooked by scholars treating the social aspects of the medieval Ashkenazi experience, provides yet another window to a better understanding of these Jews' everyday lives, values, and mentality, and to social components other than its scholarly elite.

Medical marginalia

What exactly did people record or copy in the margins and blank spaces of the manuscripts that contained the texts used by the learned elite of medieval Ashkenazi Jewry? As noted, this material is extremely varied, not only in theme and genre, but also in its paleography. The marginal notations were perhaps recorded by the original scribe or owner, however later scribes and owners made additions. This might suggest that the texts were opened, consulted, and updated. Many of these entries are of a medical nature. Some are very short and simple formulas like the one quoted earlier; others are longer and more elaborate. Some prescribe the use of non-kosher ingredients, such as a remedy for leprous sores calling for the use of lard or the use of human sperm fluid (MS Paris Bibliotheque National Heb. 1122 fol. 1r).

Another type of marginal material is purely magical in nature, for example, a formula designed to ensure the favour of a non-Jewish political authoritative figure like the one found in the earlier-mentioned MS Parma Bibliotheca Palatina 2342 on fol. 205r : 'a formula of how one can be in the ruler's grace'. As this specific entry appears often in different versions and in quite a few manuscripts, it suggests that, being fearful of such encounters; Jews employed a variety of means, among them charms, incantations, and magical spells, to guarantee a satisfactory outcome. A more domestic example of a magical formula is found on the last page of MS Cambridge Trinity College F 12 27. This manuscript contains a copy of *Sefer Haminhagim*: the book of Religious Rites and Customs by the late 14th-century Ashkenazi sage Rabbi Abraham Klausner. Among the entries on the blank left on the last page (fol. 47 r) we find a charm against the evil eye in medieval French with a Hebrew translation. The magical sentences are in French, in Hebrew characters, the instructions regarding how to administer the charm are in Hebrew.

> A charm against the Evil Eye: just as a cow licks her calf to protect it, I lick my boy (in Hebrew: Na'ar Sheli) so that he will come to no harm. And he should say this three times and lick his forehead and that is the cure.

Interestingly, the language gender roles change in the charm - the French charm refers to a woman imitating a cow who licks her calf, and the Hebrew translation retains this aspect, but

[4] In 1548 Cohen purchased it in Venice from two Italian Jewish brothers. Paleographical-philological analysis by the scholars at the Institute for Microfilmed Hebrew Manuscripts at the Jewish National and University Library in Jerusalem led to the discovery that the 'missing half' of this MS is yet another MS from the same Bibliotheca Palatina at Parma: MS Parma 2295 (Di Rossi 563).

[5] Scholarly scrutiny of these 'conventional' medieval *materia medica* requires the skills and thorough medical, philosophical, astrological and medieval-scientific knowledge displayed by the late Julius Preuss, Joshua Leibovitz, and Sussman Muntner. More recent scholarship on this matter can be founds in the works of Ron Barkai, John Efron, Shmuel Kottek, Tzvi Langerman, and Josef Schatzmiller, to name just a few. On Preuss and his work see: Rosner 1977. On the works of Joshuah Leibowitz (not to be confused with his cousin Yesha'ayahu Leibowitz) see Wilk 1985. On the works of Sussman Muntner see Muntner 1949; Muntner 1961. Ron Barkai's work is of special importance to the study of medieval Gynaecological practice and knowledge: see Barkai 1991; Barkai 1998. Shmuel Kottek wrote extensively on Jewish medical knowledge in the European Middle Ages: a partial list of his publications and scholarly interests can be found in *Korot* 9 1991, 755-766. Tzvi Langerman dedicated some of his writing to the social aspects of medieval Jewish medicine as well as the flow of scientific and medical knowledge across denominational divides: see Langerman 1996; Langerman *et al* (eds.) 2005; Langerman 2006. Joseph Shatzmiller's work re-examined some of the previous scholarship like that of Muntner's: Shatzmiller 1982; Shatzmiller 1983; Shatzmiller 1994. John Efron's work bridges the gap between the Middle Ages and the early modern and modern era: see Efron 2001. For a fine short summary of the role of Jews in medieval European medicine, see Jankrift 2004.

when the text moves to explain the instructions, the Hebrew changes from the female gender to the male. This might indicate that the French source was a feminine French popular practice, yet since it was transcribed into Hebrew, probably by a male scribe or practitioner, the gender has changed due to the recorder's gender affiliation.

In some cases the marginal entries come from what are known as 'Magical Usage Books' (*Sifrei Shimush*).[6] These were glosses written on the margins of sacred, usually biblical texts, like the book of Psalms, or the *Siddur* - the Jewish parallel to the Christian missal - containing instructions on what to do and say in order to spark divine intervention. The instructions link the recitation of a certain chapter, verse, or group of verses to a specific purpose. There usually is a thematic link between the text recited and its purpose. One such *Sefer Shimush* is found in MS Parma 2189, a 14th century Ashkenazi manuscript, containing, among other texts, the third division of the Hebrew bible the *Ketuvim* (*Psalms*, *Proverbs*, the books of *Esther*, *Ruth*, *Lamentations*, *Ecclesiastics*, *Song of Songs*, *Ezra*, *Nehemiah*, and the *Two Books of Chronicles*). In this manuscript, the uses (*shimushim*), or magical entries, appear as glosses on the margins of the book of Psalms.

The situations addressed in these entries vary, ranging from cases of minor illness to acute and debilitating disease. Other matters indicated are situations requiring luck and special need of fortune. For example the gloss on Psalm 51 reads: 'For a headache: one should recite this psalm ... three times and say: May it be your will, O living and eternal God Yahweh, to deliver me [the patient's name] from any ache or pain. Amen Amen Sela.' On Psalm 132, the gloss reads:

> 'To catch many fish: write this psalm up until the words *Tzeda Barech* (lit.: bless our game), tie it to the fishing net and many fish will be caught'. And on Psalms 110 the gloss reads: 'For a woman with difficulty in labour: write this psalm till the 3rd verse (*Ke'khadrei Kodesh Me'Rekhem*- literally: 'in majestic holiness, from the womb'), fasten it to the woman's thigh and she will deliver instantly, with God's help. To defeat an enemy say the whole psalm as if sobbing (הכובכ)'. The last example indicates that certain Psalms were used in more than one fashion, and as in many magical formulas and charms, there are specific instructions regarding the recitation of the charm to ensure its potency.

Thus far we have dealt with Hebrew material, namely formulas and instructions penned in Hebrew on the margins of Hebrew Rabbinic manuscripts. However, not all the marginal entries are in Hebrew, as we have seen earlier with the translated French magical formula. Nonetheless, even if in a language spoken by Jews other than Hebrew, the entries are written in Hebrew characters. Some are formulas that provide, alongside the Hebrew, instructions in German, Yiddish, and medieval French or Provencal. This is especially true for names of natural ingredients (mainly plants); such names were more likely to be familiar in the local vernacular. In other cases we find instructions in Judeo-languages, or in a combination of Hebrew and the vernacular, to ensure the instructions are carried out properly by those Jews whose knowledge of Hebrew was not that intimate - they could decipher Hebrew writing, but their command of the language itself was poor. This perhaps suggests that the formulas were utilized by a wider range of people than just the learned Hebrew-reading elite, the consumers of the main texts penned in the MS.

A fine example of this comes from MS Oxford Bodleian 271 (formerly Opp. 31). Between folios 87 and 89, a wide variety of practical usage entries appear, including recipes for medicines and instructions for the home production of ink, as well as of gold and silver dyes. One of these entries is a remedy for a skin disease that reads: '...And the rest should be poured on his head, he means: *ober sein toct* three times a day for 23 consecutive days'.

Another case where vernacular languages appear is in words to be recited orally as a charm or spell designed to enhance the remedy's effect. These words were recited either while carrying out the treatment or later. In some cases we see the strong influence of the surrounding non-Jewish society, as in this suggested cure for a childless woman found in MS Oxford Bodleian Library 641 (Ox. Bodl. 641; Opp. Add. Fol. no.034) fol. 81v:

> A treatment for a barren woman. She should take a ...[and here follows a list of ingredients and specified quantities] and she should cook them with good strong wine in a large firm metal pot. And while the pot is still piping hot she should sit on the pot and do this three times a day for eight consecutive days so that the scent will penetrate her body through the uterus to warm the placenta. And then she should take her menstrual blood and place it in a vessel with some water. If she wishes to have a male child she should go to a pear tree and kneel before it as night turns to day and say to the tree: *Birnbaum , ich klage Gott und dir dass mir ist genommen meine Frucht gif (=gib) mir deine Frucht und nimm meine un-Frucht.*[7] And she should pour her menstrual blood on the tree and repeat this for three consecutive mornings when night ends and day begins and then she should take a piece of the tree and cook it with water and take a male child's navel [i.e. the remains of the navel cord] and crush it in the water and drink it.

The formula goes on to provide the reader with a similar remedy for bearing a female child. In that case the woman should turn to an apple tree (*Apfelbaum*) and recite a similar text. The formula just quoted appears in a blank between two Jewish legal works along with other medical remedies for leprosy and skin diseases. The obvious pre-Christian pagan nature of the text is apparent; however it did not prevent the scribe or the owner from recording it between two texts that represent a culture which we would have thought to be opposed to magical machinations of this specific nature (appealing to trees and nature deities).

[6] The use of the words of the Holy Scripture, deemed sacred for their divine origin, for the purpose of magical healing predates the Middle Ages and can be traced to Roman Palestine. See: Hezser 2001, 209-226. However the format discussed here (*Sifrei Shimush*) is a medieval construct that probably dates back no earlier than the early Islamic period (7th-10th century).

[7] 'Pear tree! I protest to God and to you for my fruit has been taken from me. Give me your fruit and take away my infertility'.

Let us take a closer look at this entry. It provides a fine example of the eclectic nature of some of the 'household' remedies penned on the margins of rabbinic manuscripts. The Oxford MS, like similar ones discussed earlier, is a typical 14th century Ashkenazi rabbinic manuscript. It was recently described in full detail by Simcha Emanuel because it contains a relative abundance of important Jewish legal material, from the writings of Rabbi Meir of Rothenburg. Needless to say the recipe I have just quoted does not appear in Emanuel's description. Apparently, the formula quoted was recorded because people either used or thought of using it and because they believed it might actually be effective, just like the other, less 'spicy' material found written in the same hand on that page. Furthermore, it seems that whoever copied the formula did not see any contradiction between its rather obvious pagan origin and features and the main texts found in the MS in close proximity. The Talmudic ruling: 'whatever is used as a remedy is not [forbidden] on account of the ways of the Amorite' (Babylonian Talmud tractate Shabbat. 67a) probably paved the way for such a permissive attitude.

This recipe combines two separate bodies of medieval medical knowledge. Greco-Roman Hippocratic and Galenic medical traditions concerning female anatomy resonate strongly in its first part. The method of having warm vapours and steam penetrate the uterus was not uncommon and was often prescribed for gynaecological problems as early as the 3rd century BC.[8] However, the second half of the procedure is even more remarkable. It bears a striking resemblance to texts of a similar nature recorded and analyzed nearly a century ago by German scholars in the *Handworterbuch des Deutschen Aberglaubens* (The Encyclopaedia of German Superstition) published in Berlin in the late 1920s.[9] Folklorists since Frazer have designated the appeal to the pear and apple trees, and the method of exchange exemplified by the formula, as sympathetic magic.[10] In Germanic, Celtic and Norse pre-Christian cultures of Europe, tree magic was a well-established body of knowledge: the apple tree and the pear tree were, like many other trees, thought to harbour magical qualities, and are much referred to as being of special importance in these cultures.[11] These methods, common among the pre-Christian Germanic and Celtic inhabitants of Western Europe, were, as Stephen Wilson noted, found in this region during the High Middle Ages, the early modern era, and even into the late 19th and early 20th centuries.[12]

What is a recipe from a pre-Christian magical tradition doing in between two rabbinic legal texts? First of all, let me point out that this phenomenon is not unique to Jewish manuscripts. Yitzchak Hen, an expert on Medieval Latin liturgical texts from the Franco-German environment, brought its occurrence in numerous medieval Christian manuscripts of a canonical-liturgical nature to my attention. Texts of a magical, sometimes-pagan nature were inserted in the margins or in between texts containing Christian sacred liturgy. Although many examples attest to this phenomenon, one suffices to strengthen the point made here. MS Florence, Biblioteca Medicea-Laurenziana, Ashburnham 82 (32), fol. 16v-17r contains some formulae for divination and prodigies scribbled into some blank spaces and on the margins, not long after the original text of the codex was copied. The manuscript itself is a canonical-liturgical manuscript intended to assist a priest (!) in the execution of his pastoral duties.[13] Turning back to the Hebrew manuscript, it seems that the copier of this formula saw no reason not to use it and apparently no contradiction between its nature and the nature of the rabbinic material copied on the adjacent folios. It further indicates the exchange of domestic medico-magical knowledge that was a common practice in medieval Europe in what appears to be much wider circles then once assumed.[14]

The final example to be discussed brings us full circle to the manuscript with which this paper began. In view of the last entry discussed, which was strongly influenced by the surrounding non-Jewish society, it is interesting to find an entry of an opposite nature. In the middle of the MS Parma 2343 (folios 262-267), between two much larger bodies of rabbinic material, we find a long list of various medico-magical entries designed to meet a large variety of physical, mental, and other needs. Unlike some other cases in which the scribe specified the origin of the text copied, here the origin of this list is not clear and was not specified. Nonetheless, the added-on text appears to be a properly-edited list and not just a random collection. It may have been compiled by the scribe of the manuscript himself or copied from an existing list, perhaps a Jewish physician's notebook. This last hypothesis is strengthened by the words *Bakhun u'mnuseh*, which mean 'tested and proven', written next to some of the entries, indicating that someone had systematically checked their efficacy.

The list divulges a cluster of troubling, though solvable, issues and situations for Ashkenazi Jews. The term 'solvable' is of some importance in this case. Myths surrounding magical practitioners and the image and aura promoted by fairy tales, popular literature and, more recently, motion picture culture, created the false impression of self-awareness among magical practitioners verging on omnipotence. It should be noted that those individuals who actually practiced magic in a vocational fashion, and especially magical healers, wise men and woman, and those who used magic to aid others, in many ways tended to restrict themselves to treating matters where they believed a change would actually be attributed to their intervention. The reason for this is commercial as well as a sort of disclaimer intended to disassociate their intervention from any failure.[15] But let us turn back to the list. Some of the more than 50 entries are: to bring a man from afar; to stop the flow of menstrual blood; to retrieve a man's sanity; for a man whose wife hates him; a contraceptive remedy; a potion for a child frightened at night and for children who wet their beds, etc.

The following short but puzzling remark appears next to one of the entries: 'Tested and proven, and this should not be shown to a gentile. For a man who has difficulty urinating....'.

[8] Barkai 1998, 6-68. On the use of warm vapours to 'encourage' the uterus to become fertile see: Barkai 1995.
[9] Hoffmann-Krayer and Bachtold-Staubli 1927, 519-22; 1339-42.
[10] Frazer 1922, 11-45.
[11] Balmires 1997.
[12] Wilson 2000.
[13] Hen 2001, 43-58.
[14] Shoham-Steiner 2006, 375-6.
[15] Harari 2001, 14-42.

This entry is somewhat puzzling both because Jews were well-known medical practitioners in almost every corner of the Jewish Diaspora, and because there was a constant interfaith exchange of medical knowledge throughout the Middle Ages as we have seen above. Medical know-how flowed from both sides of the religious divide. This is true not only for professional practitioners of medicine, as can be seen from the extensive translation of medical tractates from Arabic, Latin and Greek into Hebrew as well as the other way around, but it also applied to domestic neighbourly connections as well. It seems that only among extremely pious Jews, whose views are reflected in works like *Sefer Hasidim*, do we find rulings designed to limit this exchange, especially when the methods of healing involved the use of non-kosher ingredients or typically Christian folk remedies. These domestic medical connections are demonstrated by two exempla, one Jewish and one Christian, both from the turn of the 12th century.

In a moving story, the author of the 13th century *Book of the Pious* (Rabbi Judah ben Shmuel 'the Pious' of Regensburg, Germany) praises a Jewish mother for rejecting her non-Jewish neighbour's offer to use a stone relic chipped from the Church of the Holy Sepulchre in Jerusalem to heal her dying son. From the phrasing of the exemplum it is clear that the son died. I think it safe to say that *Sefer Hasidim*'s praise for this mother frames, by way of contrast, the fact that Jews indeed employed Christian relics, or methods of healing with clearly Christian origins. [16] In a Christian exemplum story from England, the mirror image of this story describes the same situation from a pious Christian point of view. In the story, a Jewish woman asks her Christian neighbour, with whom she is friendly, to stop by her house on her return from the shrine of St. Thomas Becket with a bucket of holy water obtained there. The Jewess wanted the water to heal her sore leg. According to the story, no sooner had the Christian neighbour crossed the threshold of the Jewish home, than the saint, angered by the blasphemous use of his healing powers on a heathen, miraculously caused the bucket to split into three. The water spilled out, thereby preventing either woman from using the water for a potentially miraculous cure. [17] Notwithstanding the opposition by pious circles reflected in these exempla, it appears that Jews and Christians alike exchanged domestic medical cures on an everyday basis.[18]

In the light of the above mentioned two statements, we might be able to explain the enigmatic phrase: 'this should not be shown to a gentile'. One possibility is that someone was trying to keep 'professional secrets' from a potential competitor, thus supporting the conjecture that the aforementioned list was copied from a medico-magical practitioner's notebook; the other is that the prescribed treatment was so dangerous that its failed application to a member of the outside group of 'gentiles' would have more far-reaching consequences than just an unhappy neighbour.

[16] See Wistinezki 1891, § 1552 (Hebrew).

[17] Jacobs 1893, 153.

[18] Shoham-Steiner 2006, 375-6.

Conclusions

As stated at the beginning, the phenomenon discussed here is not unknown to scholars of Jewish studies, especially those involved in deciphering medieval manuscripts. It was over a century ago that the first scholars of the *Wissenschaft des Judentums*, such as Moritz Steinschneider, Avraham Berliner, and Leopold Zunz, called our attention to it. In the first volume of his monumental trilogy *Geschichte des Erziehungswesens und der Cultur der abendländischen Juden während des Mittelalters*, Rabbi Moritz Güdemann of Vienna devoted an entire chapter (chapter seven) to what he called: 'The Belief in Magic, Sorcery, Witches and other such nonsense among Franco-German Jewry in the 12th and 13th Centuries'.

Güdemann, a typical product of the *Wissenschaft des Judentums* and the Jewish enlightenment (*Haskalah*) movements, as well as of 19th century German romanticism, had an obvious, not so 'hidden agenda' for this chapter, as well as for the other parts of his book. His purpose was to show how Jews and Christians shared common beliefs and how, despite persecution, Jews were as much a part of the medieval Franco-German cultural framework as Christians. The popular beliefs Güdeman called 'nonsense and superstition' were perfect examples of his thesis. Influenced by the teachings of the enlightenment, to Güdeman's mind it was also important to demonstrate that the cultural influence proceeded from Christians to Jews and not the other way, and that traces of these superstitions could be found in 12th- and 13th-century Jewish writings.

Güdemann laboured to show how cultural representatives of Franco-German Jewry in this period, like Rabbi Meir of Rothenburg, Rabbi Isaac ben Moshe of Vienna (compiler of the popular *halakhic* compendium *Or Zarua*), and, above all, *Sefer Hasidim* (The Book of the Pious), the work compiled by Rabbi Judah 'the Pious' of Regensburg (d.1217), exemplify Ashkenazi popular culture. This is especially true of the latter (*Sefer Hasidim*), a text Güdemann believed was a genuine representative of the collective efforts of medieval Ashkenazi culture.[19] In his mind, it was Christian and pagan 'superstition' which influenced Ashkenazi Jewry, and not the other way around. Contemporary scholars have also commented on this phenomenon. In his recently published *Peering Through the Lattices*, Ephraim Kanarfogel convincingly argues that not only German Jews (*Hasidei Ashkenaz*) but a rather wider circle of Franco-German Jewry were involved in mysticism, divination, and the occult, even in circles once thought of as 'diehard' rationalists, like the Tosafists.[20]

My aim differs somewhat from that of Güdeman and his colleagues, on the one hand, and from Kanarfogel, on the other. I think we should look not only at the authors of medieval Ashkenazi rabbinic material, namely, at the main corpus of texts, but also at those who can be labelled as consumers, owners, and users of scholarly rabbinic material. It seems that the copyists of this medico-magical and practical material were not troubled by its placement in close proximity to classic rabbinic material. In some cases, the very quantity of

[19] Güdemann 1880-1888.

[20] Kanarfogel 2000, 19-31.

material seems to indicate a strong desire to record it. It seems that most of the material described briefly here was recorded for domestic use, just as we keep headache, painkillers and cough syrup handy. It seems plausible that in serious cases, 'authorized' medical practitioners were consulted and asked to aid or heal, yet in mundane matters such a consultation would have occurred only after the marginal entries were consulted. Indeed, we know that consulting a medical authority or 'authorized' practitioner in medicine and magic in medieval Europe was at times a costly matter. A fine testimony to this effect survived in this quote from 13th-century northern France. The cost of medicine emerges in a brief quotation from a ruling by Rabbi Judah Sir Leon of Paris and Rabbi Moses of Evreux (the quotation itself is from Rabbi Moshe of Coucy's 13th century *opus magnum*, *Sefer Mitzvot Gadol*): 'Once, a man had his money stolen. He vowed to pay someone 100 *denarii* for conjuring the demons so he could identify the thief. Eventually the man refused to pay the practitioner the 100 *denars* and our Rabbi made him pay. The same is true for medicine, for it is common practice to pay a large sum for these matters'.[21]

This statement makes it clear that large fees were generally collected for medical treatment and for practical sorcery alike. This explains why learned people would have wanted to have at least some practical medico-magical knowledge at their immediate disposal. But this is not the sole reason for the appearance of this material in Hebrew Rabbinic manuscripts. Medical consultation was not the only costly aspect here: parchment, paper, and writing materials were also rather expensive commodities in medieval Europe. Only a handful of people, scholars and jurists by profession, or the wealthy, could afford a private manuscript library. In many cases the library content was no more then a handful of codices, many of which were of an eclectic nature, compiled and collected piecemeal over time.

Most of the individuals engaged in scholarly learning knew much of the essential material (Babylonian Talmudic tractates for the most part) by heart. In quite a few institutions of learning, traditions dating back to Talmudic times (4th to 7th century) instilled the notion that memorization of large portions of essential scholarly material was a prerequisite to scholarly learning. This should not surprise us, for in many cases the Jewish institutions of learning relied heavily on student knowledge and on student-owned books, and possessed no 'proper' libraries. To this we must add the fact that many of the individuals seeking to study with a well-known master had to 'hit the road' and travel, sometimes great distances, to a centre of learning of their choice. Given the conditions of travel, they naturally took along only essential books and texts.

Thus, in most medieval Ashkenazi-Jewish households where a scholar lived, the entire home library might consist of a codex or perhaps two handwritten volumes bound together. Considered part of family property, we find instances where family members seized these assets during inheritance quarrels, or in divorce cases, as seen from a late 13th-century Ashkenazi *responsum* (*Teshuvot Ha'Rosh*).[22] At times, these manuscripts or codices were the only writing material available. This explains why they were used to record or copy the 'other' non-rabbinic texts alongside the rabbinic ones. Although recipes, remedies, and magical formulas do not exhaust the types of additional material one could expect to find in a Jewish household manuscript, for me, however, they are the most intriguing. Owing their preservation to their apparently harmonious coexistence with classic rabbinic texts, I, for one, am grateful for the glimpse they provide of medieval Ashkenazi Jewry's everyday concerns and their remedies.

Acknowledgements

This article began as a lecture delivered at the 35th annual conference of the Association for Jewish Studies (AJS) in Boston on December 2003. A revised edition was presented in the 2nd *Annual International Workshop on Disease Disability and Medicine in Early Medieval Europe 400-1200* which focused on *Concepts of Health and a Healthy Body* at the University of Nottingham in July 2007. I wish to thank Sally Crawford, Ted Fram, Ephraim Kanarfogel, Christina Lee and Bernard Septimus, for sharing their insightful comments on this paper with me. Of course the responsibility for this article is mine alone.

Bibliography

Abulafia, A.S. 2004. 'Christians and Jews in the High Middle Ages: Christian Views of Jews', in C. Cluse (ed), *The Jews of Europe in the Middle Ages: (tenth to fifteenth centuries), Proceedings of the International Symposium held at Speyer, 20-25 October 2002*, 19-28, Turnhout: Brepols.

Blamires, S. 1997. *Celtic Tree Mysteries: Practical Druid Magic and Divination*, St.Paul MI: Llewellyn.

Barkai, R. 1991. *Les infortunes de Dinah: le livre de la generation: la gynecologie juive au Moyen-Age*, Paris:Cerf.

Barkai, R. 1995. 'Greek medical traditions and their impact on conceptions of woman in the gynecological writing in the Middle Ages', in Y. Azmon (ed.), *A View into the Lives of Woman in Jewish Societies – Collected Essays*, 115-142, Jerusalem. (Hebrew).

Barkai, R. 1998. *A History of Jewish Gynaecological Texts in the Middle Ages*, Leiden-Boston-Köln: Brill.

Efron, J.M. 2001. *Medicine and the German Jews: A History*, New Haven and London: Yale.

Emanuel, S. 2006. *Fragments of the Tablets: Lost Books of the Tosaphists*, Jerusalem. (Hebrew).

Frazer, J. 1922. *The Golden Bough: A Study in Magic and Religion*, New York: Macmillan.

Güdemann, M. 1880-1888. *Geschichte des Erziehungswesens und der Cultur der abendländischen Juden, während des Mittelalters und der neueren Zeit, Vol.I-III*, Wien.

[21] Rabbi Judah Sir Leon was one of the leading Talmudic scholars of his time in early 13th century northern France. Rabbi Judah was the mentor of the illustrious Rabbi Moshe of Coucy, the editor and compiler of one of the most important *halakhic* manuals of High middle Ages known as *Sefer Mitzvot Gadol* (The Large Book of Commandments). On these 13th century Rabbinic figures see: Gross 1876, 173-210; Urbach 1986, II 321-34, 465-92 and recently Emanuel 2006, 191-198, esp. 194.

[22] Shoham-Steiner 2007, 175-176.

Gross, H. 1876. 'Jeudah Sir Leon aus Paris', *Magazin für Geschichte und Wissenschaft des Judentums*, **4**, 173-210.

Harari, Y. 2001 'Power and Money: The Economical Aspects of the use of Magic by Jews in Late Antiquity and the Early medieval Period, Pe'amim', *Studies in the Cultural Heritage of Oriental Jewry,* **85**, 14-42. (Hebrew).

Hen, Y. 2001. 'Educating the Clergy: Canon Law and Liturgy in a Carolingian Handbook from the time of Charles the Bald', in Y. Hen (ed.), *'De Sion exibit lex et verbum domini de Hierusalem: Essays on Medieval Law, Liturgy and Literature in Honor of Amnon Linder*, 43-58, Turnhout: Brepols.

Hezser C. 2001. *Jewish Literacy in Roman Palestine*, Tubingen: Paul Mohr Verlag.

Hoffmann-Krayer, E. and Bachtold-Staubli, H. (eds) 1927. *Handworterbuch des Deutschen Aberglaubens, Vol. 1*, Berlin-Leipzig.

Jacobs, J. 1893. *The Jews of Angevin England: Documents and Records from Latin and Hebrew Sources*, London.

Jankrift, K.P. 2004. 'Jews in Medieval European Medicine', in C. Cluse (ed.), *The Jews of Europe in the Middle Ages (tenth to fifteenth centuries: Proceedings of the International Symposium held at Speyer, 20-25 October 2002)*, 331-339, Turnhout: Brepols.

Kanarfogel, E. 2000. *Peering through the Lattices – Mystical Magical and Pietistic Dimensions of the Tosafist Period*, Detroit: Wayne State University Press.

Langerman T. 1996. 'Fixing a cost for medical care: medical ethics and socio-economic reality in Christian Spain as reflected in Jewish sources', in S.S. Kottek and L. García-Ballester (eds), *Medicine and medical ethics in medieval and early modern Spain: an intercultural approach*, 154-162, Jerusalem: Magnes Press.

Langerman T. *et. al.*, eds, 2005. *Hebrew medical astrology: David Ben Yom Tov, Kelal qatan: original Hebrew text, medieval Latin translation, modern English translation*, Philadelphia: American Philosophical Society.

Langerman T. 2006. 'Medical "Isra'iliyyat"?: Ancient Islamic medical traditions transcribed into the Hebrew alphabet', *Aleph*, **6**, 373-398.

Malkiel, D. 2007. 'Jews and Apostates in Medieval Europe: Boundaries Real and Imagined', *Past and Present*, **194**, 3-34.

Muntner, S.B. 1949. *The Book of Medicine by Asaph*, New York.

Muntner, S.B. 1961. *The History of Medicine: Sexology in the Bible and Talmud*, Lisbon.

Rosner, F. 1977. 'Julius Preuss: The father of Hebrew medical research', *Leo Baeck Institute Year Book*, **22**, 257-269.

Shatzmiller, J. 1982. 'Doctors and Medical Practices in Germany around the year 1200: The Evidence of Sefer Hasidim', *Journal of Jewish Studies*, **33**, 583-593.

Shatzmiller, J. 1983. 'Doctors and Medical Practices in Germany around the year 1200: The Evidence of Sefer Asaf', *Proceedings of the American Academy for Jewish Research*, **50**, 149-164.

Shatzmiller, J. 1994. *Jews, Medicine and the Medieval Society*, Berkeley-Los Angeles: University of California Press.

Shoham-Steiner, E. 2006. '"For a prayer in that place would be most welcome": Jews, Holy Shrines and Miracles – a new approach', *Viator*, **37**, 369-395.

Shoham-Steiner, E. 2007. *Involuntary Marginals: Marginal Individuals in Medieval Northern European Jewish Society*, Jerusalem (Hebrew).

Skinner, P. 2003. 'Confronting the "Medieval" in Medieval History: The Jewish Example', *Past and Present*, **181**, 219-247.

Urbach, E.E. 1986. *The Tosaphot - Their History, Writings and Methods (5th expanded edition), Vol. I-II*, Jerusalem (Hebrew).

Wilk, D. 1985. 'Prof. J.O. Leibowitz - bibliography (1933-1984)', *Korot*, **8**, 7-23.

Wilson, S. 2000. *The Magical Universe: Everyday Ritual and Magic in Pre-Modern Europe*, London.

Wistinezki J., ed. 1891. *Judah b. Shmuel 'the Pious': Sefer Hasidim*, Berlin. (Hebrew).

Chapter Seven

Asclepius, Biographical Dictionaries, and the transmission of science in the Medieval Muslim world

Keren Abbou Hershkovits

Introduction

The history of science in the Muslim world is a dynamic field that is in a phase of changing focuses and new approaches. Various issues are being re-examined. In this article I would like to address one of these issues. I will reconstruct and analyze the attitude(s) of Muslim scholars toward scientific knowledge and activity. I hope to show how scholars used the biography of Asclepius, whose knowledge was derived partly from prophecy, for an elaboration of their understanding of what the sources of science were. This reconstruction was approached through biographical dictionaries devoted specifically to scientists. Their places and times of production were limited to 10th-century Al-Andalus and 12th- and 13th-century Syria and Egypt. I hope to show that viewing these attitudes as part of constant (and in some cases violent) struggle is a distorting approach. I chose bibliographical dictionaries for several reasons. A first reason is that they dedicate space to discussing not only the people, but also the process of transmission of science in general to Muslim scholars.[1] As a consequence, they include a discussion of the origins of scientific knowledge within their biographies, usually at the very beginning of the dictionary in the first few entries. Another reason for this choice is that their authors did not declare their book to be a defence of the sciences (such as Ibn Rushd's *Tahāfut al-tahāfut*). Nor were they a direct response to criticism against science, but a delivery of the author's opinion regarding science and its cultivation. A third reason is that science is at the centre of these books. While there are dictionaries which mention philosophers or men of science among others, the dictionaries which are the focus of this paper are dedicated strictly to men of science.

This period of the Umayyad Caliphate in al-Andalus, and the Ayyūbid and Mamlūk periods in Egypt and Syria, has been under re-examination in the past few years. We have difficulties in assessing the attitude toward science and men of science in the context of the late phase of the Umayyad Caliphate in al-Andalus. It is now clear those previous assumptions, arguing that the sciences were rejected for religious reasons, should be questioned and re-considered.[2]

Similarly, the current state of scholarship in the field of the history of science in the Ayyūbid and Mamlūk periods has no clear and definite statements regarding the prevailing attitude toward the cultivation of science. Until the 1990s it was usually argued that the *ulamā* and the practitioners of science were in constant struggle. However, recent scholarship (as will be demonstrated below) has shown the limited character of our picture in relation to the scope of scientific activity in this period. Likewise, we do not fully understand what the nature of the interaction between scholars was, or of that between scholars and rulers.

Rulers' attitudes toward science are also currently being questioned and re-examined. For instance, Michael Chamberlain's study covers the 12th and 13th centuries in Damascus and 'address[es] the relations among power, culture and social life in a more general level'.[3] One of the themes examined was the interactions between rulers and scholars, including several attempts of rulers to set the tone in terms of what would be studied or not. Chamberlain's main conclusion was that in the high medieval Middle East neither the state nor a religious body held power, but rather the élite household.[4]

According to Chamberlain, the *a*ᶜ*yān* (notables) of Damascus appreciated knowledge in many forms, including medicine, mathematics, theology, and *belles-lettres*. Chamberlain demonstrates that during the 12th to 14th centuries, education was very pluralistic. He presents several incidents of teachers in Damascus who are known to have taught various sciences, including philosophy, natural sciences and medicine, and they kept their teaching position at *madrasahs* nonetheless.[5] Chamberlain also argues that when rulers attempted to direct the program of study, these attempts often failed.[6] According to Chamberlain, the dismissal of teachers and the criticism against particular educational programs should be studied as a part of a struggle among intellectual élites looking to preserve or increase their power, rather than as disapproval of the cultivation of science. Rulers could not impose a chosen doctrine in the *madrasahs*, the program was determined by the teachers themselves.

In her study of Ayyūbid and early Mamlūk Damascus, Sonja Brentjes makes similar arguments. Brentjes examined incidents generally claimed to be examples of rulers' and scholars' disapproval of the cultivation of science. One such incident is al-Āmidī's (1156-1233) dismissal from his post as a teacher in the ᶜAzīziyya *madrasah* in Damascus in 1229. It was commonly agreed by modern scholars that the reason for this

[1] 'Science' in this context means the disciplines considered by the authors of the dictionaries, i.e. medicine, the mathematical sciences, natural philosophy, logic, metaphysics and logic.

[2] Monès 1998 51-85. See also the introduction to this book, esp. pp. xix ff.

[3] Chamberlain 1994, 7.

[4] *Ibid* 2.

[5] *Ibid* 171-175.

[6] *Ibid,* 84-87.

dismissal was al-Āmidī's interest in philosophy and science.[7] Brentjes examined several versions of al-Āmidī's biography and showed that the various biographies present different reasons for his dismissal. Each biography portrays a different person. She argues that some of the biographies do not agree with the claim that al-Āmidī's misfortune was the direct result of his interest in science. Her main conclusion is that we should not read anecdotes of dismissal, prosecutions, executions and accusations at face value. Rather, we should look into the context within which the anecdotes were written and carefully examine each source for variations and contradictions. These variations will reveal that most accusations were the result of personal disagreements or professional rivalry, rather than a strict rejection of science or philosophy.[8]

There were probably some points of disagreement, tensions, and perhaps animosities among scholars; the nature of these rivalries deserves further study. Such a study will determine what part the cultivation of science played in these rivalries. The real reason for arguments, persecutions and so on, is not the important issue to look for. What should be examined is how the descriptions and presentations of such debates and rivalries reflect norms and values of people, groups and communities. If one wishes to learn about the intellectual milieu in these periods, one needs to study the social practices of the elite, and to examine the various locations where studies took place.

Furthermore, David King has shown that the current state of research does not reflect the range of scientific activity taking place under the Ayyūbids and Mamlūks in the field of astronomy.[9] Similar arguments were raised by Leigh Chipman regarding medicine and pharmacology, and Housni al-Khatib-Shechadeh has demonstrated the same for veterinary medicine.[10] Therefore, there is no clear picture as to how and to what extent the sciences were actually cultivated under the Ayyūbids and Mamlūks.

Until such a study is conducted, clear and decisive arguments about the attitude toward science under the Ayyūbids and Mamlūks will be problematic. Consequently, I will not make arguments regarding the context. Rather, I will try to present the authors' perspective: what they wrote about science, and suggest explanations for the biography each created/transmitted. Through this presentation I wish to address the question of attitude through texts which demonstrate a positive and inclusive approach toward science. This kind of reading fits into current scholarship that downplays struggle and conflict between religion and science.

Biographical dictionaries are a unique Islamic genre, dedicated to the biographies of people belonging to a defined group: viziers, poets, jurists, blind people, teachers of a specific *madhhab*, inhabitants of a certain city etc. Such dictionaries were written in the Muslim world starting from the 9th and up to the 19th centuries.[11] Biographical dictionaries usually follow a rather strict formula; an entry usually starts by describing the correct way to pronounce the name; date of birth; a genealogy; lists of teachers and pupils; and finally, note books that the subject of the biography composed/translated/commented upon.[12] Sometimes the author of the dictionary would add anecdotes about the person, or mention whether his works received some kind of re-examination (e.g. if somebody corrected or commented upon his treatise).

Several biographical dictionaries were dedicated to practitioners of science. They appeared between the 10th to the 13th centuries, in various geographic regions. Some were dedicated to a particular branch of science, while others were more general and include scholars of all sciences. The most famous are *Kitāb tabaqat al-attibā'* by Ibn Juljul (944 - post 1009, in al-Andalus),[13] *Ikhbar al-'ulamā' fī akhbar al-ḥukamā'* by Ibn al-Qifṭī (1172 - 1248, in Aleppo),[14] and *'Uyūn al-anbā'* by Ibn Abī Uṣaibi^cah (1203 - 1270, in Cairo).[15]

These dictionaries reflect the fascinating process of the naturalization and appropriation of foreign knowledge in the Muslim world. This process was first brought to the attention of researchers of Islamic sciences by A.I. Sabra, who argued that once scientific texts were translated, the knowledge contained in them was transformed. The text, its contents and sometimes even the uses of the knowledge, were changed to fit the needs and interests of Islamic culture.[16] According to H.A.R. Gibb, the information presented in biographical dictionaries demonstrate the authors' concept that: 'the history of the Islamic Community is essentially the contribution of individual men and women to the building up and transmission of its specific culture; that it is these persons... who represent or reflect the active forces in Muslin society in their respective spheres; and that their individual contributions are worthy of being recorded for future generations'.[17] The inclusion of people in dictionaries is an indication that the authors perceived them and their cultivation of science as having been personally responsible for the creation of Islamic society. Hence, as I will later argue, biographical dictionaries should be read as a part of a narrative presenting scientific knowledge and its sources as an integral part of any Islamic community, a narrative that was written by Muslim scholars writing in different genres, times and places. By discussing Asclepius and recounting his biography, the authors appropriated his figure into a Muslim world, and explain his importance for the whole community.

The authors of the above-mentioned dictionaries lived in different times and places, yet, as I will demonstrate below, they should be viewed as a part of a network of scholars discussing the framework within which science can be cultivated. In this I

[7] Humphreys 1977, 209; Sourdel 1971, 434.

[8] It should be noted however, that the very use of cultivation of science as a point of criticism indicates that the issue of the cultivation of science was under debate, or a point of tension.

[9] King 1983. See also: Charette 2003, 9.

[10] See Chipman 2009. In addition, there is an abundant material in chronicles waiting to be recorded and analyzed (I thank Dr. Housni al-Khatib Shechade for bringing this to my attention).

[11] On biographical dictionaries, their character and the information stemming from this genre see: Rosenthal 1968; Young 1990; al-Qāḍī 1995; Young 2006.

[12] Gibb 1962.

[13] Ibn Juljul in Fuad Sayed 1955. On the author, see Dietrich 1971, 755.

[14] Ibn al-Qifṭī in Lippert 1903. On the author, see Dietrich 1971, 840.

[15] Ibn Abī Uṣaib^cah in Niẓar Riḍā 1965. On the author, see Vernet 1971, 693.

[16] Sabra 1987, 223-43. See also Jamil Ragep's analysis of Sabra's article in Ragep 1996, xvii.

[17] Gibb 1962, 54.

follow Randall Collins' theory of the sociology of philosophy. One of his arguments is that an idea or a theory should be examined not only in light of its historical context, but also in relation to the network within which it was presented and practiced. Such networks can be reconstructed by investigating which authors quoted one another, and referred to each other. The consideration of similar themes, theories and ideas are another way to identify a network. I am using the term 'network' in Collins' diachronic sense.[18]

The Andalusian judge and physician Ibn Juljul was the personal physician of al-Muʾayyad bi-Allāh Hishām (r. 976 - 1009). He dedicated his dictionary to physicians (or at least people whose fame was mainly due to their medical knowledge). The first person he mentions is Hermes, the fourth figure is Asclepius. The first four biographies form a narrative of the transmission of science and its first cultivation by humans.

Ibn al-Qifṭī, a judge and administrator in Aleppo, wrote about all the sciences, including arithmetic, astronomy, philosophy, medicine, and astrology. He mentions Ibn Juljul as one of his sources, cites significant parts his dictionary, and summarizes parts of it. In addition, they both refer to similar medical and historical texts (such as Galen's or Hippocrates' texts, or Abū Maʿshar's *Kitāb al-ūluf*). Ibn Abī Uṣaibiʿah (hereafter IAU), a physician, and the head of the Nūrī hospital in Damascus and the Nāṣirī hospital in Cairo, quotes both Ibn Juljul (IJ) and Ibn al-Qifṭī (IQ), mentions them by name, and again refers to similar previous sources.

The three share several common features (in addition to the interest in the life of scholars). One of these commonalities was their interest in the question: who was the first person to engage in science and how did he acquired his knowledge? The first few biographies suggest a narrative of the transmission of science to Muslim scholars, and its sources.[19] Though each dictionary has its own unique organization, each author structures the whole text in such a way that the story of science is dealt with first. Though I will not use other texts in this article, it is of importance to see that the three biographical dictionaries do not stand alone, but that there are other texts of different genres dealing with similar subjects.[20] All these texts can be viewed as a part of the same network of scholars, scholars who discussed the status of scientific knowledge and of the practitioners of science vis-à-vis other intellectual activities and pursuits.

One of the names repeatedly appearing in these dictionaries as a source for medical knowledge is that of Asclepius. The biographies attributed to Asclepius in these dictionaries shed light on how the origin of medicine was perceived. As I will show below, the analysis of Asclepius' biography informs us how scholars constructed the narrative of the transmission of science. It reveals their hidden (or not so hidden) agendas as well as their constraints and tools. In addition, it uncovers their ideas regarding the cultivation of science, its sources, legitimacy, and targets.

The Biographies

Asclepius' biographies differ in size and the inclusion or exclusion of information. However, there are several issues that were addressed by all three authors. In what follows I will discuss similarities, differences and their meanings. The following information appears in all three texts:

a. Asclepius cultivated medicine;

b. The sources of his knowledge and his teachers;

c. His knowledge was acquired through inspiration;[21]

d. God acknowledged Asclepius as an angel: 'Galen has mentioned that God has inspired [*awḥā*] Asclepius. [God said] I would rather call you "an angel", as it describes you better than "human"';[22]

e. Asclepius never died but ascended to the heavens while still alive: Hippocrates wrote that '[He] was raised to the sky in a column of light';[23]

f. Asclepius was a role model of moral behaviour, and God-fearing.

The three authors mention Asclepius as a physician and an important one. All three dedicate a significant part of the biography to a discussion regarding the sources of his knowledge; I will begin by examining the suggestions appearing in each dictionary.

Sources of Knowledge

It was generally accepted that Asclepius was the first, or one of the earliest, humans to cultivate medicine. The sources of his knowledge and the identities of his teachers were one of the major issues all three dictionaries dealt with. According to all three dictionaries, Asclepius had a teacher, but he was also granted with inspiration, and even God-given inspiration. The three authors used two terms for the word 'inspiration': *ilhām* and *waḥy*. There is a difference between these two terms. The noun *ilhām* is generally used for inspiration in general, while *waḥy* (from the verb *awḥā)* denotes specifically divine inspiration. It is usually used in the context of the revelation of the Qurʾān to Muḥammad and other prophets.[24]

The authors differ, though, with regard to teachers. Ibn Juljul mentions Hermes the Egyptian as Asclepius' teacher. The biography of Hermes the Egyptian precedes Asclepius', describing the fields of knowledge he specialized in (poisons, the nature of lands and others), and time of life (after the Flood). However, Ibn al-Qifṭī and Ibn Abī Uṣaybiʿah argued that the source was another Hermes, also known as Idrīs:

[18] Collins, 2000; Collins 1989.

[19] The description of a chain of transmission to scientific knowledge could be an allusion to an Islamic religious concept according to which religious norms and idea should be traced back to the sayings of the Prophet Muḥammad. I hope to pursue this examination elsewhere.

[20] For instance: the introduction of al-Shaharazūrī's *Nuzat al-arwāḥ wa-rawḍat al-afrāḥ*, ed. Amin ʿUthmān, in: *Nuṣūṣ Falsafiya*, Cairo, 1976. Or narratives that can be found in several of al-Bīrūnī'd treatises.

[21] *ilhām* and *waḥy*, IJ p. 9; IQ p.9; IAU p. 30

[22] IJ p.10; IQ p. 9; IAU p. 30

[23] IJ p.10; IQ p. 9; IAU p. 30

[24] On the difference between Ilhām and awāha see: MacDonald 1971, 1119. See IJ p. 10; IQ p. 9; IAU p. 30.

'Asclepius was one of four kings who accompanied Hermes and learnt from him [*akhadhū ᶜanhu al-ḥikma*]'.[25]

At this point the reader is referred to another biography, that of Hermes, where he is informed that Hermes was actually Idrīs, the mysterious Qurᵓānic prophet.[26] It is further argued that the prophecy of Idrīs included knowledge of the sciences. Medicine was part of Idrīs' prophecy of the sciences. The biography illustrates the characteristics of Idrīs, his knowledge, and how he delegated authority upon his death. Asclepius is mentioned as one of four disciples, each of whom was assigned a quarter of the earth to rule as a king, and given specific knowledge. As his disciple and successor in ruling and teaching, Asclepius held responsibilities and knowledge that originated from prophecy. The knowledge taken from Hermes/Idrīs comes in addition to the inspiration Asclepius himself received from God.[27] IQ adds to Asclepius' roles the role of a king, a leader of a community, and not only the role of the provider of medical knowledge to people. This role places Asclepius in a similar position to the disciples of the Prophet Muḥammad who were at the same time both the transmitters of the Prophet's saying, and designated leaders of the Islamic Community.[28]

The unique interaction with God does not end with divine inspiration. It is also argued that God gave him the title 'angel' instead of 'human' [*inna allāh awḥā ilā asqalībiyūs [...] an usammiyaka malakan aqrab minka an usammiyaka insānan*]. In addition, Asclepius never died; rather, he was raised up to the skies in a column of light. Asclepius is credited with a special honour which very few ever received (apart from the prophets Elijah and Idrīs/Enoch),[29] ascending to heaven while still alive. Thus Asclepius is put into the same category as these two prophets. A human being dies and goes to heaven (hopefully), therefore, since Asclepius never died, his humanity is contested and questioned and he seems to be in some kind of intermediate position: between human and angel. Furthermore, the idea of light has great importance in Islamic religious thought. Light is related to the light of guidance, prophecy and a mark of prophets. The ascendance of Asclepius in a column of light could be an additional reinforcement of his being an important figure, guided by heavenly light.[30]

Characteristics

All three authors attributed the following qualities and behaviour to Asclepius: he is God-fearing, preached people to take what the good God bestows and not to ask for more, and to conduct a moral life. These traits are not only mentioned but also demonstrated through several anecdotes. This description is followed by several anecdotes, in one of which Asclepius was worshipping [*mushtāghalan bi-ᵓl-taqdīs*], when a couple entered the shrine. They were worried about the foetus the woman was carrying. Asclepius told them that she would give birth to a *jīnn*, as punishment for their behaviour.

As shown by Nimrod Hurvitz, anecdotes serve as a means to demonstrate and strengthen the readers' understanding of the subject's traits and conduct. In his study of Ibn Ḥanbal's biographies, Hurvitz shows that the anecdotes, which seem to be out of place at first glance, are actually a tool to create affiliation between Ibn Ḥanbal and the Prophet Muḥammad's way of life.[31] Following Hurvitz' suggestion, I will argue that these anecdotes all present Asclepius as a moral person, a guide for the community, and as preaching against wrongdoing (or prophesying punishment for such behaviour).

IJ and IQ make an effort to explain the moral derived from the anecdotes:

> Hippocrates explains the meaning of the name Asclepius and that Asclepius did not like teaching but those who followed his way [*sīra*] of purity, were virtuous and God-fearing [*al-ᵓafāf wa-'l-taqī*]. He did not like teaching [medicine to] the wicked [*shirār*] and the loathsome ones [*dhū al-nafs al-khabīṭa*]. Asclepius preferred those who studied [medicine] to be the honourable [*ashrāf*] and those who acknowledged God [*mutaᵓalahūn*], that is, those who know God Almighty. It is necessary that the man of medicine [*'ālim 'ilm al-ṭibb*] be merciful, modest and like helping others.[32]

The qualities ascribed above to Asclepius fit the Islamic model of appropriate behaviour. Though Ibn Juljul did not claim medicine to be revealed knowledge, his description of Asclepius sheds unique light on the science of medicine. Asclepius is described as a pious, moral and pure person. By depicting the first person to cultivate medicine in this way, piety and purity are attributed to the science itself. A Muslim reader could identify with the figure portrayed and appreciate Asclepius' personality as well as his knowledge.

Asclepius is portrayed in religious-Islamic terms and as having his own way (*sīrah*) of purity, an allusion to Muḥammad's *sīrah* (biography, way of life). All the traits mentioned – humility, piety, morality, staying away from evil, and fear of God – are usually attributed to religious scholars. In this way, the authors create an affiliation between physicians and religious scholars, the study of medicine and the study of religion. This assumption is further corroborated by Ibn Juljul's concluding remarks: 'All the sources I have quoted earlier demonstrate that the beginning of medicine and philosophy was in revelation and God-given inspiration'.[33] Here it is clear that the author wishes to create affiliation between the science of medicine and other kinds of knowledge, particularly religious knowledge, thereby justifying the pursuit of science.[34]

---

[25] IQ p. 8; IAU p. 30

[26] IQ begins his dictionary with a short introduction, explaining his motivations and intentions in writing the dictionary and arranged his book alphabetically. The first biography cited is Idrīs/Hermes. Therefore, when the reader reads Asclepius' biography he is already familiar with the name and characteristics. IAU has a different order, in which the biographies are arranged chronologically and geographically. Idrīs' biography appears right after the claim that he was Asclepius' teacher.

[27] The identification of Idrīs and Hermes and his unique character deserves its own study. For further information on Idrīs and his identification with Enoch and Hermes see: Alexander 1998; Erder 1990; Plessner 1954; Fowden 1986, 24ff.

[28] See for instance: Madelung 2010. See also: Crone 2004, 286ff.

[29] On the identification of Idrīs with Enoch see Erder 2009, 484: Erder 2009.

[30] For light and its relation to prophecy and a mark of prophets see: Rubin 1975.

[31] Hurvitz 2003.

[32] IJ p. 11; IQ p. 9.

[33] IJ p. 13.

[34] At this point it might be worth comparing the *ṭibb al-nabī* (prophetic

Why should these authors, all important and well-respected figures in their time, take the trouble to describe Asclepius in such terms? What were their motivations? Was it necessary? Or were they perhaps continuing ancient traditions of describing physicians in general to Asclepius in particular? The following will be my attempt to answer these questions.

The suggested similarities between the medical and religious scholars might be a reference to the words of al-Shāfiʿī (the founder of the Shāfiʿī school of law, d. 820): 'There are two kinds of knowledge: the science of religion [*dīn*] which is *fiqh*, and the study of the bodies, which is medicine'.[35] It is possible that the presentation of the sources of medicine as divine inspiration alludes to al-Shāfiʿī's saying. However, none of the authors mention either al-Shāfiʿī, or his words explicitly.

Another possibility is that the authors continued earlier concepts related to Asclepius. According to Yulia Ustinova, already at the dawn of Greek history, by the 8th century BC, Asclepius was considered to have supernatural healing powers. He was one of several historical or semi-historical figures who had exceptional interactions with the gods and healing powers.[36] By the 5th century BC, his mortal status was changed to immortal. From that time onward, Asclepius was considered the god of healing and was worshipped as such in sanctuaries. His mortal worshippers were visited by him in their dreams, and as a consequence, learned how to treat a medical situation.[37]

Though it is possible that Muslims were following and continuing earlier depictions of Asclepius, this explanation still seems incomplete. The current state of scholarship does not allow us to determine to what extent 10th to 13th century scholars were familiar with ancient concepts of Asclepius, which of the texts was translated, and what each author read. This point deserves some further study. However, the very concept of dismissing Asclepius' image in biographical dictionaries as nothing but following in the footsteps of the ancients is problematic. Even if Muslim authors were familiar with ancient biographical information, their transmission of this information and creation of new meanings for each category (such as what 'superhuman' meant and what can be considered 'healing power' or proper conduct) is new and deserves its own study. So does the very choice of including these anecdotes and descriptions in their biographies. Thus, I would argue that the answer (or at least part of the answer) should be searched for in the wider context of the transmission and appropriation of Greek science in the Muslim world.

Asclepius and Socrates

Asclepius is not the only ancient non-Islamic figure portrayed as pious.[38] Another interesting case is the figure of Socrates as depicted in Arabic literature. In a comprehensive study, Ilai Alon unfolds the reasons for the attention Socrates received from Muslim scholars. According to this study, the main reason was the fact that Socrates could be presented to Muslim readers as teaching both ethical and philosophical lessons. Similarly to the prophet Muḥammad, whose *sīrah* should be studied, as well as his divine message, Socrates was considered to be a law giver, using the Arabic term *sharāʾiʿ* (religious law) and leading the proper life.[39]

There are other parallels between Socrates and Muḥammad, as well as other religious figures. For instance, Socrates is called 'the seal of mystical wisdom', this time an allusion to the Prophet Muḥammad, who was called 'the seal of the prophets'. He thought of this world as a bridge to the next world, and he appreciated piety and overcoming one's lust. Some Muslim scholars even argued that Socrates actually was a prophet. Ibn Sīnā, the famous physician, is one example.[40]

Socrates appears in the 'Mirror for Princes' genre as a model of good behaviour for rulers. Muslims shared this appreciation of Socrates, and he was referred to as 'al-ḥakīm al-muta'allih' (the deistic philosopher, metaphysician or theologian).[41] Some of the quotes related by Socrates are attributed elsewhere to King David, Jesus, the prophet Muḥammad, Abū Bakr (the first caliph) and others.[42] In addition, Socrates played an important role as a legitimating authority in religious controversies between rationalist Muslims and more traditionalist scholars. The fact that Socrates' life and sayings could be seen as alluding to those of the prophet gave the rationalists' arguments more credibility and weight.[43] Thus, argues Ilai Alon, the use of Islamic-religious terms was a means to present Socrates to an Islamic audience as a role model for appropriate moral behaviour.[44] Both Socrates' actions and sayings are in conformity with Islamic religion or can be connected to Islam. Socrates' sayings use Islamic terms such as idols (*aṣnām*), or polytheism (*shirk*) and the improvement of character (*taḥdīd al-akhlāq*), which suggest similarities between Socrates and Abraham.

---

medicine) genre, where medical treatment is based on Muḥammad's sayings. Irmeli Pehro examined the development of this genre, and argued that its aim was "to transfer the medical authority from Galen to the Prophet. But ... not to discard Galen or deny the merits of Graeco-Islamic medicine. ... an attempt to bring forth a new form of medicine, that would combine Islamic teachings and Graeco-Islamic medical theory" (Perho 1995, 78). The most structured texts dealing with the medicine of the prophet date from the later part of the 13th and the 14th centuries, a period later then that of the texts being examined in this paper. For the development of this genres, its sources and motivations see: Perho 1995 53ff.

[35] Al-Shāfiʿī's remark was directed to prophetic medicine. Cited in: Bürgel 1976 56.

[36] He was called "the blameless physician", see: Edelstein and Edelstein 1998 2, 2ff. Ancient scholars, such as Cicero and Xenophon mentioned Asclepius, his knowledge and his deification. The reason given for the immortalization of Asclepius, is his teaching of medicine to humans. For quotes from Greek sources regarding Asclepius' divine nature, see: ibid, 1, 108-178.

[37] See: Ustinova 2002; Ustinova 2004.

[38] Examples can also be found outside the field of science and scholars as well. For instance, Deborah Tor demonstrates that ancient Iranian rulers were portrayed as role models for proper Islamic religious conduct (Tor forthcoming). Tor shows that Muslim scholars and chronicles relate Islamic characteristics to ancient Iranian figures, and attributed the moral behavior expected from a Muslim to them. One of the most interesting examples is Niẓām al-Mulk's presentation of Anūshīrvān (a famous Sasanian ruler, d. 579) as a role model for proper religious behaviour. I thank the author for allowing me to read a draft of the article.

[39] Alon, 1991, 88.

[40] See Alon 1991, 11 for other prominent Muslim figures who discussed Socrates and his religious qualities. See *ibid,* 92 for modern Muslim scholars' appreciation of Socrates.

[41] Alon 1991: 87.

[42] Alon, *Socrates,* 87-91.

[43] Socrates was looked upon with religious eyes from antiquity and well into the 12th century, both by Christians and Muslims. Khomeini for instance called Socrates 'a great theologian' (Alon 1991, 92).

[44] Alon 1991.

The figure of Asclepius, as presented by biographical dictionaries, has much in common with the characteristics attributed to Socrates. They were both pious, conducted a moral life, and demanded that others follow their example. It seems the motivation was the same in both cases: the desire to present a foreign figure to the Islamic community in such a way that their foreignness would be less conspicuous. Another aim was to make Asclepius's knowledge (and that of Socrates, too, for that matter) acceptable to the Islamic community. By presenting the sources of Asclepius's knowledge as legitimate and by portraying him as ethical and pious, his knowledge of medicine could be considered legitimate and worthy. The reader of these three biographical dictionaries is left with the understanding that medicine originated in divine inspiration, if not in straightforward prophecy. Moreover, physicians (as followers of Asclepius) are viewed as standing on the same plane as religious scholars, holding the same values, following the same way of life and cultivating knowledge which originated in the same source, i.e. the divine.

The attitude expressed by the authors can also be understood through the differences between them. One difference has already been mentioned. IJ argues that Asclepius' teacher was Hermes the Egyptian, while IQ and IAU wrote that it was Idrīs who taught medicine (and more) to Asclepius. The reason for this difference is not clear; it is possible that IQ and IAU, who copied extensive parts from IJ, made a mistake.[45] However, this possibility is not very likely. IAU ascribed the information regarding Asclepius' teacher to another source:[46] Abū Ma'shar al-Balkhī (d. 886).[47] IQ quotes IJ at the end of the biography, and explains that Hermes, also known as Idrīs, lived in Upper Egypt. This might have been the root of the confusion between Hermes/Idrīs and Hermes the Egyptian.

Another interesting difference is the title given to Asclepius by IQ: Asclepius al-ḥakīm – Asclepius the Wise. IQ titles only two people 'al-ḥakīm': Asclepius and Luqmān. IQ is very careful in his use of words, he does not use the title *ḥakim* for physician in general, but in these two cases only. Such a choice links the two figures of Asclepius and Luqmān. Luqmān the Wise is mentioned in the Qur'ān (31: 12). He is considered a person who chose wisdom over prophecy. Arabic literature of all genres, including religious and historical, acknowledges Luqmān as a wise person, though his exact identity is debated.[48] His unique and outstanding wisdom and piety allowed him to be included in the genre of 'Tales of the Prophets' (*qiṣaṣ al-anbiyāʾ*), though he was not a prophet.[49] IQ's usage of the title *ḥakim* for both is another way to familiarize Asclepius and to connect him with figures well known in Islamic religious literature.

IQ has the longest biography of the three. The main reason for that is that he added information not directly related to Asclepius' life. One example is that he quotes the Hippocratic Oath.[50] Another reason is that IQ and IAU also quote the *Fihrist* of Ibn al-Nadīm. This source is missing from IJ's dictionary.[51] As this text has been widely studied I will only refer to it very briefly. The *Fihrist* (*The Catalogue*) was written between 987-8, in Baghdad. Ibn al-Nadīm has several narratives describing the transmission of science in general, and medicine in particular, to the Muslim world. However, Asclepius plays only a small role in these narratives. Ibn al-Nadīm merely mentions his name as the first of eight important physicians in history. But he does not elaborate on the sources of Asclepius' knowledge, nor on the quality of his knowledge.

Ibn al-Nadīm states that the source of his information regarding the beginning of medicine was Isḥāq Ibn Ḥunayn's (d. 910) treatise.[52] Both authors acknowledge Yaḥyā al-Naḥwī as their source.[53] The first part of Isḥāq's treatise deals with the question of the origins of medical knowledge. However, there is no one final conclusion; rather the author suggests several options. Isḥāq wrote that Asclepius was the first to 'discuss some aspects of medicine'. According to Isḥāq, Asclepius's knowledge was partially invented by him, and partially received by experience. Isḥāq further argues that experience is not considered a human activity, but God's way of intervening in the world: 'Others say that God gave medicine to mankind through inspiration by experience'.[54] One wonders why Ibn al-Nadīm does not elaborate on this point.[55] However, reading the whole chapter about the sciences reveals that Ibn al-Nadīm is very consistent in arguing that science is a human invention and practice. Ibn al-Nadīm cites several narratives of sciences; all of which put man (a person or a nation) at the centre of the cultivation of science.[56]

Though both IQ and IAU quote Ibn al-Nadīm's version of Isḥāq ibn Ḥunayn's treatise, they end up with a very different description of Asclepius's role in transmitting and teaching medicine to humans. The order of the information given changes the way the reader relates to the text. IQ and IAU first establish the sources of Asclepius's knowledge (i.e. God-given inspiration and Idrīs's revelation), and only then do they turn to quote Ibn al-Nadīm. Thus, when the reader reads the story of eight important physicians, with Asclepius being the first of them in IQ and IAU, he already knows where the knowledge came from. Ibn al-Nadīm does not provide such information,

[45] It is accepted that Ibn Abū Uṣaybiʿah copied significant parts from Ibn al-Qifṭī. See Vernet 1971.
[46] IAU in Nizar Rida 1965, 30.
[47] Burnett 2009.
[48] Masʿūdī, for instance, wrote that there is no person as wise and pious as Luqmān. (Masʿūdī 1966, 1, 63f sec. 105). For a medieval survey of the various anecdotes related to Luqmān see Brinner 2002, 586.
[49] Heller and Stillmann, 2009.
[50] IQ p. 9.
[51] Dodge, 572-576. For a short biography see: Fück 1971. Ibn al-Nadīm was the son of a bookbinder in Baghdad. Very little information is available regarding his life. Most of the details we do know come from his book. See also Stewart 2007, 369-387. In this article, Stewart analyses the order and organization of the text as a means to reveal al-Nadīm's concept of Islamic sciences. The *Fihrist* has a chapter on science and men of science but is not dedicated to the sciences.
[52] The text was extensively studied by Franz Rosenthal: Rosenthal 1954, 55.
[53] The figure of Yaḥyā al-Naḥwī is ambiguous. Very little is known about him, and most of it is contradictory. Some say that he lived in Alexandria, in the 6th century, while others claim that he lived in the 7th century. He is usually identified with Joannes Gramatikos. See: Meyerhof 1930.
[54] Rosenthal 1954, 63 (English translation p. 74). 'Ta'rīḫ al-Aṭibbā' appears also in other biographical dictionaries, including the ones being analyzed in this paper. For the variations between the different versions see: *ibid.* 61-71.
[55] As al-Naḥwī's original text is now lost, there is no way to determine what the original claim regarding the divine help Asclepius did or did not receive was.
[56] Al-Nadīm 2: 272ff.

and the reader of Ibn al-Nadim alone cannot tell where the first physician drew his knowledge from. This is an example of how the same text can serve different agendas. While Ibn al-Nadīm presents the sciences, medicine included, as a human creation and activity, other dictionaries argue differently, and wish to present medicine as part of the religion-related branches of knowledge.

Narratives of Transmission

Medicine was a part of a wide corpus of scientific knowledge translated into Arabic, starting from the second half of the 8th century.[57] In the course of the translation and transmission of scientific texts and knowledge,[58] that knowledge underwent a process of transformation. The cultivation of science originating outside the realm of Islam brought many problems, religious as well as technical, to the fore. Therefore, the texts and scientific theories were appropriated and transformed in their new cultural context, producing new cultural artefacts.[59]

Transmission and transformation include changes in the contents of the texts. These changes were sometimes the result of linguistic constraints, but also of cultural and religious needs and difficulties. For instance, the Hippocratic Oath mentions various deities, and the Arabic translation includes Apollo's name, but not as a deity, as in the Greek text, but rather as a great teacher or physician. Other deities appearing in the Oath were omitted and Allah took their place.[60] Another problem was the introduction of medicines derived from ingredients that were unsuitable for Muslims, such as wine or unclean animals, or plants that were unavailable to inhabitants of the region.

However, scholars had to face a more basic question: does knowledge that originated in pagan nations have any value for Muslims?[61] How should one approach the study of such sciences? Narratives of science are an attempt to address these and other issues. Moreover, they are both the result and a part of the process of transformation. The story of science needed to be invented, reinvented and transformed to fit into the culture of Islam. The various narratives found in medieval Islamic literature reflect the values that were important for each author (and for his contemporaries?) and reveal the discourse that scholars took part in at particular points in time. These narratives were a part of scholars' definition of their place in society, and a means to situate their kind of knowledge within the intellectual (and social) network of their times. Such narratives appear in various genres: biographical dictionaries, chronicles, professional (scientific) texts and philosophical texts. Narratives of science situate the knowledge of medicine vis-à-vis other kinds of knowledge. They act as a definition of medical science while shaping and conceptualizing *what* is science or knowledge.

I would argue that the three biographical dictionaries examined in this paper are an arena for discourse regarding the position of medicine and the origin of medical knowledge. The authors of these dictionaries had no argument with previous scholars who granted Asclepius the honour of being the first, or one of the first, to practice medicine. However, it was not clear to them who he actually was, and what the sources of his knowledge were. The narrative depicted in the biographies aims to elucidate and explain these ambiguities. Such an assumption could also explain IJ's remark: 'This is the information I found regarding Asclepius that seems to be rational. There are other stories [related to him] in Christian historical books, but they are not found in our book'.[62] The other issue is the need to situate Asclepius, and the knowledge attributed to him, in a legitimate position. The construction of his biography depicts the construction of contemporary concepts regarding the value of knowledge and of legitimate sources of knowledge. By attributing to Asclepius the particular characteristics mentioned above, and by presenting him as the first or one of the first to cultivate medicine, the authors made a statement regarding medicine, i.e. Asclepius being pious, pure and God-fearing, qualifies him as a reliable source for medical knowledge. Pagan connotations are replaced by familiar Islamic ones.

Therefore, this presentation of Asclepius could be considered an attempt to integrate medicine, its concepts and its practitioners, into a legitimate Muslim world. It is not a cynical manipulation, or a well-calculated forgery, it is the writing of Muslim scholars, thinking in Islamic terms, perceiving themselves as part of that world, rather than outsiders. These authors wrote from and for an Islamic society, a society shaped to some extent by religious role models. Thus the use of religious terminology is not surprising. Authors of various genres adopted *ḥadīth* forms and used the Qurᶜān and Muḥammad's sayings as a means to prove their information was reliable. Authors of biographical dictionaries used similar literary tools (for instance, the use of religious terminology and the construction of Asclepius's figure according to accepted ideas of a religious role model).[63]

Biographical dictionaries were not the only genre to present a narrative of science. As mentioned, Ibn al-Nadīm, whose book belongs to a slightly different genre - bio-bibliography - illustrated the cultivation of medicine as a human activity. Such a notion appears also in other narratives, which were not included in this paper. Further study is needed to determine the reasons for this difference, i.e. science as a human creation versus science as revelation (biographical dictionaries focus on the person whereas the bio-bibliographic dictionary focuses more on the books produced/available). These two attitudes are of significant importance as to the understanding of how science should be practiced. These attitudes also have implications

[57] A recent study by George Saliba has questioned this assertion, arguing that the first translations were done already during the late 7th century. Moreover, Saliba argues that the Arabs in the Arabian Peninsula had much more sophisticated knowledge than commonly believed. See Saliba 2007, introduction.

[58] For a description and historical analysis of the translation movement, see Gutas 1998.

[59] Scott 2003, 4.

[60] For other examples see: Pormann and Savage-Smith, 2007, 32-33; Ullmann, 1978, 30-31.

[61] See for instance the following cases: Heck, 2006; Livingstone 1992; Mahd 1970; Zysow 1984, 291; or the Hanbalī scholar Ibn Taymiyya's attitude in: Street 2005.

[62] IJ p. 12: *fahadhā mā wajadtuhī madūnā min akhbār Asqālibios alqarībah min alma'qūl. Walahu akhbār fi twaārīkh alnaṣārī shanī'ah lā yutlīq bikitābunā.*

[63] Khan 1969.

for concepts such as the possibility of change and progress in scientific knowledge. If science is revealed knowledge, not only is it legitimate, but it is necessary to cultivate science as part of an Islamic way of life. But, if science is a human creation, a new set of assumptions and questions arises; what made this creation possible? Does God approve it? How can we differentiate between legitimate scientific knowledge and illegitimate knowledge? Can revealed knowledge be critiqued? Expanded? Improved?

Both notions, i.e. science as a human creation, or science as part of a prophecy, appeared already by the 10th century, and were repeatedly mentioned up to the 14th century. Both notions were presented in different geographical and political contexts by people who were also courtiers. It would seem possible that the two explanations are an outcome of two networks of scholars, networks that need to be further studied and explored.

Summary

Throughout its history, Islamic society has been engaged in a dynamic debate regarding inclusion and exclusion of norms, values, knowledge and so on. The debate regarding what is 'new (*bidᶜa*), and therefore illegitimate, is a good example of that. In a way, the question of the legitimacy of science is a part of this debate. By presenting medical knowledge as divine or partly divine, the authors of biographical dictionaries attribute legitimacy to the sources of knowledge and remove the suspicion of possible heresy. Moreover, they set a criterion for legitimate knowledge; knowledge is reliable if the sources can be traced back to prophecy or a prophet. The analysis of three of Asclepius's biographies demonstrates that the authors viewed medicine as part of revealed knowledge. Their construction of the narrative of the transmission of medicine is a possible source for modern scholars to learn what the prevailing attitudes toward science and knowledge were. They constructed the figure involved in the cultivation of medicine (and practicing it) according to this guideline. Therefore, Asclepius was guided by God, and studied under one of God's prophets - Idrīs. The portrayal of Asclepius according to religious norms and values demonstrate what the authors (and possibly their contemporaries as well) considered the important values. One can only assume that the authors of these biographical dictionaries conceived revealed knowledge to be the appropriate source for knowledge, including medical knowledge. Further study is needed to examine the way this concept, i.e. medicine and prophetic knowledge, fits into other concepts of scientific knowledge.

Acknowledgments

This paper is partly based on a chapter from my dissertation, submitted to the Senate of Ben-Gurion University, supervised by Nimrod Hurvitz; it is a great pleasure to thank him for his careful reading and wise comments and support along the way. I would also like to thank Sonja Brentjes, Faith Wallis, Leigh Chipman and Zohar Hadromi-Alluoch for reading earlier drafts of this paper and making invaluable comments. All mistakes remain my own.

Bibliography

Alexander, P. 1998. 'From Son of Adam to Second God', in M. Stone and T. Berggren (eds) *Biblical Figures outside the Bible*, 87-122, Harrisburg: Trinity Press.

Alon, I. 1991. *Socrates in Medieval Arabic Literature*, Leiden: Brill.

Brinner, W.M. (ed. and trans.) 2002. *ᶜArāʾis al-Majālis fī Qiṣas al-Anbiyāʾ or 'Lives of the Prophets' as Recounted by Abū Isḥāq Aḥmad Ibn Muḥammad Ibn Ibrāhīm al-Thaᶜlabī*, Leiden: Brill.

Bürgel, C.J. 1976. 'Secular and Religious Features of Medieval Arabic Medicine', in C. Lesley (ed.), *Asian Medical Systems: A Comparative Study*, 44-62, Berkeley, Los-Angeles: University of California Press.

Burnett, C. 'Abū Maᶜshar', *Encyclopaedia of Islam, III,* online edition accessed 14 September 2009.

Chamberlain, M. 1994. *Knowledge and Social Practice in Medieval Damascus, 1190-1350*, Cambridge: Cambridge University Press.

Charette, F. 2003. *Mathematical Instrumentation in Fourteenth-Century Egypt and Syria, the Illustrated Treatise of Najm al-Dīn al-Mīṣrī*, Leiden: Brill.

Chipman, L. 2009. *The World of Pharmacy and Pharmacists in Mamlūk Cairo*, Leiden: Brill.

Collins, R. 1989. 'Toward a Theory of Intellectual Change: The Social Causes of Philosophies', *Science, Technology and Human Values*, **14(2)**, 107-140.

Collins, R. 2000. *The Sociology of Philosophies: A Global Theory of Intellectual Change*, Cambridge MA: Belknap Press.

Crone, P. 2004. *God's Rule Government and Islam*, New York: Columbia University Press.

Dietrich, A. 1971. 'Ibn al-Kifti', in P.J. Bearman, T. Bianquis, C.E. Bosworth, E. van Donzel and W.P. Heinrichs *et al.*, *Encyclopædia of Islam, 2nd Edition, vol III*, 840, Leiden: E. J. Brill.

Dietrich, A. 1971. 'Ibn DJuldjul', P.J. Bearman, T. Bianquis, C.E. Bosworth, E. van Donzel and W.P. Heinrichs *et al.*, *Encyclopædia of Islam, 2nd Edition, vol III*, 755, Leiden: E. J. Brill.

Dodge, B. (trans) 1970. *The Fihrist of al-Nadīm: A Tenth Century Survey of Muslim Culture*, 2 vols, New York: Columbia University Press.

Edelstein E. and Edelstein, L. 1998 repr. *Asclepius Collection and Interpretation of Testimonies*, 2 vols, Baltimore: Johns Hopkin University Press.

Erder, Y. 1990. 'The Origin of the Name Idris in the Quran: A Study of the Influence of Qumran Literature on Early Islam', *Journal of Near Eastern Studies*, **49(4)**, 339-350.

Erder, Y. 2009. 'Idrīs', in J. Dammen McAuliffe (ed.), *Encyclopaedia of the Qurʾān*, 2, 484, Leiden: Brill.

Fowden, G. 1986. *The Egyptian Hermes, a Historical Approach to the late Pagan Mind*, Cambridge: Cambridge University Press.

Fuad Sayed (ed.) 1955. Ibn Juljul, *Ṭabaqāt al-Aṭibbāʾ*, Cairo: French Bureau Publications.

Fück, J.W. 1971. 'Ibn al-Nadīm', in P.J. Bearman, T. Bianquis, C.E. Bosworth, E. van Donzel and W.P. Heinrichs *et al.*, *Encyclopædia of Islam, 2nd Edition, vol III*, 895-898, Leiden: E. J. Brill.

Gibb, H. 1962. 'Islamic Biographical Literature', in B. Lewis and P.M. Holt (eds), *Historians of the Middle East*, 54-58, Oxford: Oxford University Press.

Gutas, D. 1998. *Greek Thought, Arabic Culture: The Graeco-Arabic Translation Movement in Baghdad and the Early 'Abbasid Society (2nd-4th/8th-10th Centuries)*, London: Routledge.

Heck, P. 2006. 'The Crisis of Knowledge in Islam I: The Case of al-ᶜĀmirī', *Philosophy East and West*, **56(1)**, 106-135.

Heller, B. and Stillmann, N.A. 'Lukmān', in P. Bearman, T. Bianquis, C.E. Bosworth, E. van Donzel and W.P. Heinrichs (eds), *Encyclopaedia of Islam*, on-line edition, Brill, accessed on 14 September 2009.

Humphreys, S. 1997. *From Saladin to the Mongols: the Ayyubids of Damascus 1193-1260*, Albany: State University of New York Press.

Hurvitz, N. 2003. 'From Scholarly Circles to Mass Movements: The Formation of Legal Communities in Islamic Societies', *The American Historical Review*, **108(4)**, 985-1008.

Khan, M.S. 1969. 'Miskawaih and Arabic Historiography', *Journal of the American Oriental Society*, **89(4)**, 710-730.

King, D. 1983. 'The Astronomy of the Mamluks', *Isis*, **74(4)**, 531-555.

Lippert, J. (ed), 1903. Ibn al-Qifṭī, *Taʾrīkh al-Ḥukamāʾ* Leipzig: Dieterich'sche Verlagsbuchhandlung.

Livingstone, J. W. 1992. 'Science and the Occult in the Thinking of Ibn Qayyim al-Jawziyya', *Journal of the American Oriental Society*, **112(4)**, 598-610.

MacDonald, D.B. 1971, 'Ilhām', in P.J. Bearman, T. Bianquis, C.E. Bosworth, E. van Donzel and W.P. Heinrichs *et al.*, *Encyclopædia of Islam, 2nd Edition, vol III*, 1119, Leiden: E. J. Brill.

Madelung, W. 'Imāma', in P. Bearman , Th. Bianquis , C.E. Bosworth, E. van Donzel and W.P. Heinrichs (eds), *Encyclopaedia of Islam, Second Edition*, Brill Online, Mc Gill University, accessed 22 February 2010.

Mahdi, M. 1970. 'Language and Logic in Classical Islam', in G. von Grunebaum (ed), *Logic and Islamic Culture*, 51-83, Wiesbaden: Otto-Harasowitz.

Masᶜūdī, 1966. *Les prairies d'or*, B. de Meynard et P. de Courteille, Paris: ed. Societé Asiatique.

Meyerhof, M. 1930. 'Joannes Gramatikos (Philoponos) von Alexandria und die Arabische Medizin', *Mitteilungen des Deutschen Institute für Ägyptisch Alterumskunde in Kairo*, **2**, 1-21.

Monès, H. 1998. 'The Role of Men of Religion in the History of Muslim Spain up to the End of the Caliphate', in M. Fierro and S. Julio (eds), *The Formation of Al-Andalus, part 2: Language, Religion, Culture and the Sciences*, 51-85, Aldershot: Varorium.

Niẓar Riḍā (ed.) 1965. Ibn Abī Uṣaibiᶜah.*ᶜUyūn al-anbāʾ fi-ṭabaqāt al-aṭibbāʾ*, Beirut: Dār Maktabat al-Hayāh.

Perho, I. 1995. *The Prophet's Medicine, Studia Orientalia*, Helsinki: The Finnish Oriental Society.

Plessner, M. 1954. 'Hermes Trismagistus and Arab Science', *Studia Islamica* **2**, 45-59.

Pormann, P. and Savage-Smith, E. 2007. *Medieval Islamic Medicine*. Washington: Georgetown University Press.

Al-Qāḍī, W. 1995. 'Biographical Dictionaries: Inner Structure and Cultural Significance', in G. N. Atiyeh (ed), *The Book in Islamic World: The Written Word and Communication in the Middle East*, 93-122, New York: State University of New York Press.

Al-Qāḍī, W. 2006. 'Biographical dictionaries as the scholars' alternative history of the Muslim community', in G. Endress (ed), *Organizing Knowledge: Encyclopaedic Activities in the Pre-Eighteenth Century Islamic World*, 23-75, Leiden: Brill.

Ragep, J. and Ragep, S. (eds), 1996. *Tradition, Transmission, Transformation proceedings of two conferences on the Pre-Modern Held at the University of Oklahoma*, Leiden: Brill.

Rosenthal, F. 1954. 'Isḥāq b. Ḥunayn's Ta'rīh al-Aṭibbā', *Oriens*, 7, 55-80.

Rosenthal, F. 1968. *A History of Muslim Historiography*, Leiden: Brill.

Rubin, U. 1975. 'Pre-existence and Light: Aspects of the Concepts of Nūr Muḥammad', *Israel Oriental Studies*, **5**, 62-119.

Sabra, A.I. 1987. 'The Appropriation and Subsequent Naturalization of Greek Science in Medieval Islam', *History of Science*, **25**, 223-43.

Saliba, G. 2007. *Islamic Science and the Making of the European Renaissance*, Cambridge MA: MIT Press.

Scott, M. 2003. *Science in Translation*, Chicago: University of Chicago Press.

Al-Shaharazūrī 1976. *Nuzat al-arwāḥ wa-rawḍat al-afrāḥ*, in Amin'Uthmān (ed), *Nuṣūṣ Falsafiya*, Cairo.

Sharpe, W. D. 1964. 'Isidore of Seville: The Medical Writings. An English Translation with an Introduction and Commentary', *Transactions of the American Philosophical Society*, New Series, **54(2)**, 1-75.

Sourdel, D. "al- Āmidī," in P.J. Bearman, T. Bianquis, C.E. Bosworth, E. van Donzel and W.P. Heinrichs *et al.*, *Encyclopædia of Islam, 2nd Edition, vol I*, 434, Leiden: E. J. Brill.

Stewart, D. 2007. 'The Structure of the *Fihrist*: Ibn Al-Nadīm as Historian of Islamic Legal and Theological Schools', *International Journal of Middle East Studies*, **39**, 369-387.

Street, T. 2005. 'Logic', in P. Adamson and R. C. Taylor (eds), *Cambridge Companion to Arabic Philosophy*, 247-265, Cambridge: Cambridge University Press.

Tor, D. (forthcoming). 'The Long Shadow of Pre-Islamic Iranian Rulership: Antagonism or Assimilation?' in T. Bernheimer and A. Silverstein (eds), *Late Antiquity: Eastern Perspectives*, Oxford: Oxbow.

Ullmann, M. 1978. *Islamic Medicine*, Edinburgh: Edinburgh University Press.

Ustinova, Y. 2002. 'Either a Daimon, or a Hero, or Perhaps a God: Mythical Residents of Subterranean Chambers', *Kernos*, **15**, 267-288.

Ustinova, Y. 2004. 'Truth Lies at the Bottom of a Cave: Apollo Pholeuterios, the Pholarchs of the Eleats, and Subterranean Oracles', *La Parola del passato*, **59**, 25-44.

Vernet, J. 1971. 'Ibn Abī Uṣaybiᶜa', in P.J. Bearman, T. Bianquis, C.E. Bosworth, E. van Donzel and W.P. Heinrichs *et al.* (eds), *Encyclopædia of Islam, 2nd Edition*, Leiden: E. J. Brill.

Young, M.J.L. 1990. 'Arabic Biographical Writing', in *Religion, Learning and Science in the Abbasid Period*, ed.

M.J.L.Young, J.D. Lathman and R.B. Serjeant, 168-187, Cambridge: Cambridge University Press.

Zysow, A. 1984. 'The Economy of Certainty: an Introduction to the Typology of Islamic Legal Theory', unpublished PhD thesis, Harvard University, Cambridge, MA.

www.ingramcontent.com/pod-product-compliance
Lightning Source LLC
Chambersburg PA
CBHW061305270326
41932CB00029B/3477
9781407307145